CAROLE REE

C000138694

EGYPTIAN MEDICINE

SHIRE EGYPTOLOGY

Cover illustration
Carpenters making a catafalque. A workman is having his arm examined
(top right) whilst another screams as a hammer falls on to his foot (top left).
A further workman applies eye paint to a colleague's eyes (bottom left).
Facsimile painting by Norman de Garis Davies
from the tomb of Ipuy, Deir el-Medina, Nineteenth Dynasty.
(Courtesy of the Metropolitan Museum of Art, New York, 30.4.116.)

British Library Cataloguing in Publication Data:
Reeves, Carole.
Egyptian Medicine. —
(Shire Egyptology Series; No. 15).
I. Title. II. Series.
932.
ISBN 0-7478-0127-4.

Published in 2001 by
SHIRE PUBLICATIONS LTD
Cromwell House, Church Street, Princes Risborough,
Buckinghamshire HP27 9AA, UK.
(Website: www.shirebooks.co.uk)

Series Editor: Barbara Adams.

Number 15 in the Shire Egyptology series.

ISBN 0 7478 0127 4.

First published 1992; reprinted 2001.

Printed in Great Britain by
CIT Printing Services Ltd,
Press Buildings, Merlins Bridge, Haverfordwest, Pembrokeshire SA61 1XF.

Contents

Acknowledgements

It is my privilege to extend acknowledgement to the many individuals and institutions who offered guidance, encouragement and practical assistance during the production of this book. Long before it began, however, I was drawn into an appreciation of the history of medicine by John L. Thornton, former Librarian to St Bartholomew's Hospital Medical College, whose extensive knowledge of medical history fired my imagination. It is to him that I owe an incalculable debt.

My thanks extend to the libraries, universities and museums who have allowed me to use illustrations from their collections and to Barbara Adams and Angela Thomas for their advice and criticism. Most of the line drawings have been specially prepared by Helena Jaeschke (Archaeoptyx Archaeological Drawing Services) and I proudly acknowledge her assistance. David Burder took many of the splendid photographs which appear in the book. Acknowledgement is made to W. J. Murnane and Penguin Books Limited for permission to reproduce the chronology.

List of illustrations

Chronology

From W. J. Murnane, *The Penguin Guide to Ancient Egypt*, 1983, and including names of those rulers mentioned in the text.

Neolithic Period	before 5000 BC	Fayum A
Predynastic Period	*c.*5000 - 3300 BC	
Protodynastic Period	*c.*3300 - 3050 BC	
Early Dynastic Period	3050 - 2613 BC	3050 - 2890 Dynasty I *Horus Aha (Athothis)* *Horus Djer* 2890 - 2682 Dynasty II 2686 - 2613 Dynasty III *2668 - 2649 Djoser*
Old Kingdom	2613 - 2181 BC	2613 - 2498 Dynasty IV *2589 - 2566 Khufu* *2558 - 2532 Khaefre* *2532 - 2504 Mycerinus* 2498 - 2345 Dynasty V *2491 - 2477 Sahure* *2375 - 2345 Unas* 2345 - 2181 Dynasty VI *2278 - 2184 Pepi II*
First Intermediate Period	2181 - 2040 BC	2181 - 2040 Dynasties VII-X 2134 - 2060 Dynasty XI (Theban)
Middle Kingdom	2040 - 1782 BC	2060 - 1991 Dynasty XI 1991 - 1782 Dynasty XII *1897 - 1878 Sesostris II*
Second Intermediate Period	1782 - 1570 BC	1782 - 1650 Dynasties XIII and XIV (Egyptian) 1663 - 1555 Dynasties XV and XVI (Hyksos) 1663 - 1570 Dynasty XVII (Theban)

New Kingdom	1570 - 1070 BC		
		1570 - 1293	Dynasty XVIII
		1518 - 1504	*Tuthmosis II*
		1504 - 1450	*Tuthmosis III*
		1498 - 1483	*Hatshepsut*
		1453 - 1419	*Amenophis II*
		1419 - 1386	*Tuthmosis IV*
		1386 - 1349	*Amenophis III*
		1350 - 1334	*Amenophis IV (Akhenaten)*
		1336 - 1334	*Smenkhkare*
		1334 - 1325	*Tutankhamun*
		1293 - 1185	Dynasty XIX
		1293 - 1291	*Ramesses I*
		1291 - 1278	*Seti I*
		1279 - 1212	*Ramesses II*
		1212 - 1202	*Merneptah*
		1193 - 1187	*Siptah*
		1185 - 1070	Dynasty XX
		1185 - 1182	*Sethnakhte*
		1182 - 1151	*Ramesses III*
		1145 - 1141	*Ramesses V*

Third	1070 - 713 BC		
Intermediate		1070 - 945	Dynasty XXI
Period		945 - 712	Dynasty XXII
		828 - 712	Dynasty XXIII
		724 - 713	Dynasty XXIV

Late Period	713 - 332 BC		
		713 - 656	Dynasty XXV (Nubian)
		664 - 525	Dynasty XXVI
		570 - 526	*Ahmose II*
		525 - 404	Dynasty XXVII (Persian)
		525 - 522	*Cambyses*
		521 - 486	*Darius I*
		404 - 399	Dynasty XXVIII
		399 - 380	Dynasty XXIX
		380 - 343	Dynasty XXX (Egyptian/Persian)

Graeco-Roman	332 BC - AD 395		
Period		332 - 30	Ptolemies
		205 - 180	*Ptolemy V*
		51 - 30	*Cleopatra VII*
		30 - AD 395	Roman Emperors

Byzantine Period AD 323 - 642

Islamic Period AD 642 - 1517

1
Introduction

Research into the medicine and diseases of ancient Egypt involves the study of many aspects of its civilisation. The study of literary sources and artistic representations in painting and sculpture, as well as the examination of skeletal remains and mummies, has yielded a wealth of material. In addition, the wider interaction between ancient disease and the contemporary environment involves the studies of architecture and town planning, clothing, nutrition, agriculture and animal husbandry, commerce and travel.

Medicine is both an art and a science. The art of restoring and preserving health is as old as life itself but the science of discovering and analysing the process of disease is little more than a century old and could not have been accomplished without parallel advances in technology. Modern medicine is greatly assisted by diagnostic techniques such as radiography, computed tomography, electron and light microscopy, serology and endoscopy, all of which have been applied to ancient Egyptian remains. It is now possible not only to blood-group mummies but to extract DNA by molecular cloning, to analyse trace elements in teeth by atomic absorption spectrometry, to measure metal levels in bone by X-ray fluorescence and to computerise all these details into the International Mummy Data Base held at the Manchester Museum.

The application of modern techniques to the study of Egyptian remains has enabled new diagnoses to be made and, in some cases, the old ones to be redefined. During the 1960s, for example, extensive radiological examination of a series of mummies revealed skeletal evidence of a very rare inherited disease called alkaptonuria, which deposits a characteristic black pigment into the spine. This pigment was seen in almost a quarter of the mummies X-rayed, although in modern society alkaptonuria occurs in only one person in five million. Expert papers were written which offered explanations for this remarkably high frequency of alkaptonuria in ancient Egypt. Twenty years later, a new technique called nuclear magnetic resonance spectroscopy demonstrated a molecular similarity between the black spinal pigment and juniper resin — an embalmer's material.

This book is not simply a history of Egyptian medicine. It is an attempt to present an overview of health and disease in ancient Egypt and to outline important developments in the practice of medicine. Hypothetical or unsubstantiated data have not been included but evidence from modern scientific research has been quoted where this reinforces pathological and epidemiological findings. A volume of this size can serve only as an introduction to the fascinating subject of Egyptian medicine. Interested readers will find the bibliography (chapter 8) a useful source of further information.

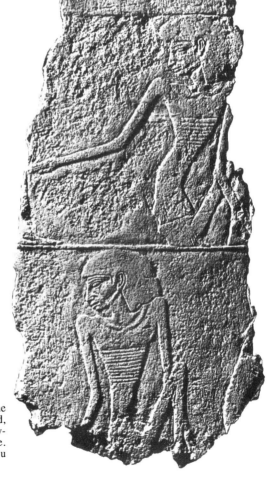

1. Limestone relief from the causeway of Unas' pyramid, Saqqara, Fifth Dynasty, showing the effects of famine. (Courtesy of the Musée du Louvre, Paris, E.17.376.)

2
Health and hygiene

During the 67-year reign of Ramesses II (Nineteenth Dynasty) an estimated 2¹/₂ million people lived in Egypt. Most were landless peasants, dependent for an existence upon the beneficence of the local landlord and the caprices of the Nile's annual inundation. When the Nile rose too high houses and fields were flooded but many times in Egypt's history the inundation proved inadequate. Lack of water brought famine, pestilence and disease (figure 1).

There are no records of how many people died during the seven-year failure of the Nile's annual flood during the reign of the Pharaoh Djoser (Third Dynasty) but it may have been many thousands. An inscription engraved on a granite block on the island of Sehel during the Greek Period tells how, during this famine:

Children wept. Grown-ups swayed. As to the old, their heart was sad, their knees gave way, they sat on the ground, their arms swinging.

The most common ordinary dwelling in early Predynastic Egypt was the round hut built of poles, reeds and mud. This was later changed to a square shape and, later still, was built of mudbricks dried in the sun — the traditional adobe house. These dwellings have survived less well than the stone-constructed tombs and temples from which much of our knowledge of ancient Egypt is derived.

During the Dynastic Period Egypt was divided into provinces, or nomes, and by the New Kingdom there were 42 nomes, each with its own administrative centre and urban development. The most densely populated areas were the Delta and the area in southern Egypt from Thebes to Aswan (estimated at over 200 people per square kilometre). Bubastis, the capital of the eighteenth nome of Lower Egypt, which was inhabited throughout the Dynastic Period, covered an area of about 75 hectares. Heliopolis, near modern-day Cairo, was the largest city in the New Kingdom and had an urban area of about 23 square kilometres.

Apart from this natural urban development there were periods when large workforces were needed for the construction of state buildings, most particularly the Pharaoh's mortuary complex. The majority of the peasant workforces used for the building of public works were employed only during the period when the Nile flooded and work on the land ceased. Remains of housing built to accommodate at least 4000 workmen have been found near the pyramid of Khaefre at Giza (Fourth Dynasty) although the maximum seasonal workforce may have numbered 100,000.

The purpose-built workmen's town of Kahun was constructed to house the officials and workforce building the pyramid of Sesostris II at Lahun in about 1895 BC. The larger houses in Kahun generally included a reception hall or living room, women's quarters, a kitchen and a room with washing or bathing facilities. There were also cellars and circular granaries. In poorer as well as rich dwellings, stone tanks used for washing were set into the mud floors, and running down the centre of every street were the remains of stone drainage channels. The town housed an estimated population of 5000 on a 14 hectare site.

Sir William Flinders Petrie, the British Egyptologist who excavated Kahun between 1888 and 1890, discovered that almost every house had been invaded by rats and their holes had been stuffed with stones and rubbish. A pottery rat trap was also found. Cats were kept to protect food and grain from rodents but, in the absence of a cat, 'cat's grease' was recommended as a deterrent.

The workmen's village of Deir el-Medina was occupied by Theban artisans for 450 years from the beginning of the Eighteenth Dynasty to the end of the Twentieth (figure 2). The dwellings were originally built of mudbrick but later housing included walls with stone bases. The single-storey, flat-roofed houses had an average of four rooms, with small windows with stone or wooden grilles. The inside walls might be decorated with frescoes or whitewashed, and wooden doors opened directly on to the street. During the reign of Seti I (Nineteenth Dynasty) there were about 600 people living in the village and, unlike in the earlier years of settlement, the animals were kept in compounds outside rather than inside the village walls.

The smallest workmen's village, at Tell el-Amarna, was built in the Eighteenth Dynasty to house the workmen constructing Akhenaten's new city, Akhetaten. It was occupied by some 350 inhabitants for about thirteen years. Each house had four areas: an outer work area, a living room, a bedroom and a kitchen with stairs leading to the roof. The houses, although not elaborate, were sturdily built with mainly whitewashed walls and ceilings.

None of these settlements had wells, so water had to be brought from the river, which, at Deir el-Medina, was over 1.5 km away. In this village water was first stored in large jars within the houses but later a community reservoir was built outside the north gate. In all the dwellings furniture was sparse and simple. People slept on the floor, on clay benches along the wall or on beds of interlaced cord with a wooden headrest. Feathers were used to stuff cushions although these were used as back supports rather than pillows.

In ordinary Egyptian homes the lavatory consisted of a wooden stool under which a cup half-filled with sand might be placed or, as at Deir

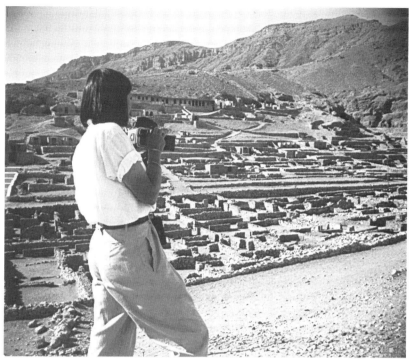

2. The remains of the workmen's village, Deir el-Medina, built to house the craftsmen who built the tombs of the Valley of the Kings, New Kingdom. (Photograph David G. Burder, FRPS.)

el-Medina, a coarse terracotta closet-stool. In the fine houses of Akhetaten bathroom suites had bath or 'shower' rooms where water was drained out of the house through a covered gully into a tank, and lavatories with wood, pottery or stone seats above large bowls of sand. All household refuse was dumped on to sites away from settlement areas.

A household commodity which would not have been wasted was food, particularly amongst poorer communities. The estimated daily intake of food during the Dynastic Period was between 480 and 576 grams, a figure comparable with that of modern Latin America. The main crops grown in Egypt were cereals: emmer wheat (*Triticum dicoccum* Shrank) for bread, and barley (*Hordeum vulgare* L.) for beer. Bread was also made from the heads of the white lotus. There were pulses such as lentils and chickpeas; vegetables such as lettuces, onions, cucumbers, leeks, radishes and garlic; fruit, particularly dates, figs, grapes and melons; plants

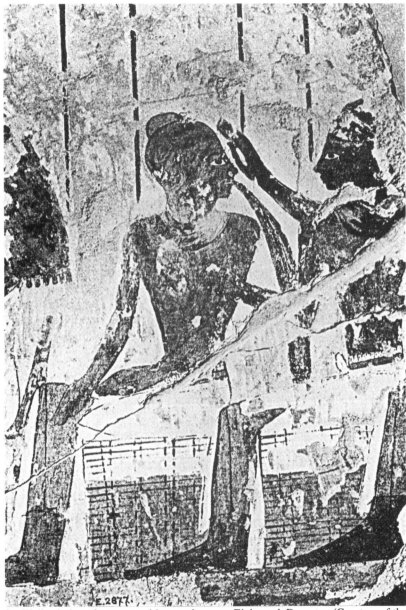

3. Wall painting of a man vomiting at a banquet, Eighteenth Dynasty. (Courtesy of the Musées Royaux d'Art et d'Histoire, Brussels, 2877.)

grown for oil, such as sesame; grapes for wine; pomegranate and palm wine were also made (the latter being used in embalming for rinsing out the abdominal cavity and washing the extracted organs); papyrus and flax for writing materials, clothing, sails and ropes. Honey, dates, raisins, 'tiger nuts' (*Cyperus esculentus* L.) and carob pods were available as sweeteners. Meat was a rare luxury for most people, herds being grazed on marginal land, especially in the marshes of the Delta. Cattle, sheep, goats and pigs were eaten. Meat, fish and fowl were dried and probably salted. Geese, ducks, quail and other game birds were fairly plentiful, and hunting these was a favourite pastime of the rich. Domestic fowl may have been a rare import during the New Kingdom but became popular in the Roman Period.

Eggs, cheese, milk and perhaps yoghurt were available. Whether milk was drunk in large quantities is uncertain. Nor is it known whether the Egyptians suffered the lactose intolerance seen in Middle Eastern and African populations today.

Most people ate three times a day even if the meal was simply bread and beer. The upper classes ate more richly if not more frequently (figure 3). Basic payment for workers and their families at Deir el-Medina was in grain, fish, vegetables and water (there was no monetary system in Egypt until the Greek Period). They also received pottery and wood for fuel. Less regular deliveries were made of cakes, beer and dates but on festive occasions bonuses were paid in salt, natron, sesame oil and meat. Clothes were occasionally supplied to supplement those woven and made in the village.

Whilst the wages were regular the community lived well but a major strike occurred in the 29th year of the reign of Ramesses III when supplies were twenty days late. The workers' protests outline the problem: 'We have come because we are hungry and thirsty. We have no clothes, we have no ointments, we have no greens.' Several more strikes occurred in successive reigns and these are the first documented instances of collective protest by a workforce.

From the 'Instruction of Duauf' (*The Satire of the Trades*, Papyrus Sallier II), written during the Middle Kingdom, we know the sort of life that the average Egyptian might expect in any trade except that of scribe, which was considered the easiest occupation of all.

I have seen the metal worker at his task at the mouth of his furnace. His fingers were like the hide of crocodiles; he stank worse than fish spawn.

The cobbler is very wretched; he is forever begging; he has nothing to bite but leather.

The fuller washeth upon the river bank, a near neighbour of the crocodiles.

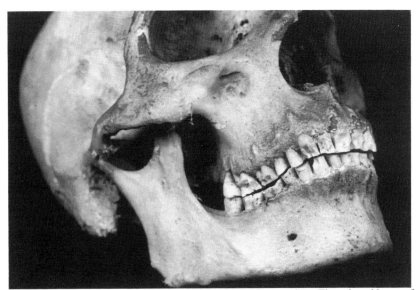

4. The teeth and jaws of a male who died in his early twenties. There is evidence of severe dental attrition. Twenty-first or Twenty-second Dynasty. (Reproduced by permission of Professor N. J. D. Smith, King's College School of Medicine and Dentistry, and Manchester University Press.)

On large building projects doctors were appointed to oversee the health of the workmen but keeping epidemic disease and occupational injuries at bay must have been an enormous task (cover illustration). A 'chief physician' was appointed for the workmen's village at Deir el-Medina and a doctor by the name of Metu was 'physician of the serfs'. There were also foremen on site who kept records on slates of absenteeism and these provide evidence of the evils keeping a man from his work. One reads: 'Fourth month of the flood day 27, Nebnefer was ill — was stung by a scorpion...'; and another: 'First month of winter day 21 Tementu was absent — had a fight with his wife...'.

There are no records of absence from work due to toothache, although most Egyptians must have suffered severely. A comprehensive study of 252 Nubian skulls spanning a ten-thousand-year period from the Mesolithic (9000 to 6000 BC) to Christian (AD 55 to 1300) eras has shown a significant reduction both in tooth size (one per cent per thousand years) and in facial masticatory musculature and proportions. A shift in diet from that of the hunter-gatherer towards carbohydrates resulted in the selection of smaller, more caries-resistant teeth, with a consequent reduction in chewing apparatus.

Of 1188 teeth examined from the Giza collection of eighteen skulls — the remains of the kinsfolk and courtiers of Pharaoh Khufu (Fourth Dynasty) — there were only 38 carious cavities. In only one instance had the cavity progressed beyond the enamel to invade the pulp chamber and cause an apical (root) abscess. The Manchester Museum collection consists of material dating from the late Dynastic, Greek and Roman Periods, where the cariogenic factor was much higher and where almost all the cavities had resulted in abscesses.

Whilst caries results in progressive loss of tooth substance and is associated with increased use of dietary sugars, periodontal disease is characterised by inflammation of the gum surrounding the tooth. Chronic inflammation eventually leads to loss of both the alveolar supporting bone and the tooth. In Egypt periodontal disease was very prevalent and was provoked by the stresses and strains applied to the teeth during chewing and by serious dental attrition (wearing down of the teeth, figure 4). 'A remedy to treat a tooth which is eaten away where the gums begin' may be found in the Ebers Papyrus. It consists of a mixture of cumin, frankincense and carob-pod pulp ground to a powder and applied to the tooth (Eb 742).

Dental attrition is common to all early populations but that seen on the teeth of almost every ancient Egyptian, throughout all periods of history, is much more extensive. Vegetables containing a high silica content, easily abraded querns for grinding corn and ill-cleansed foods are explanations common to all cultures but the Egyptians had the additional hazard of the contamination of their cereals, flour and consequently their bread by fragments of sand and by grit which may have been introduced during the milling process to act as a cutting agent. Attrition wore down the teeth to such an extent that the dental pulp became exposed and infected. This resulted in abscesses and the formation of cysts in the jaw. It also altered the shape of the cutting surfaces (cusps) of the teeth and this, in turn, caused the movements of the temporomandibular joint to become abnormal and overloaded. This eventually led to marked osteo-arthritic changes, which are very commonly seen in Egyptian skulls.

Many jaw bones show evidence of small holes, which have been interpreted as 'bore holes' made by dental surgeons to drain pus from abscesses. However, scholars such as Filce Leek have offered the alternative explanation that these holes were caused by the dissolution of the bone by pus. So numerous foci of dental infection must have undermined the health of many people and resulted in widespread halitosis. A recipe for a breath sweetener (frankincense, myrrh, cinnamon bark and other fragrant plants boiled with honey and shaped into pellets) was also used as a house fumigator.

Personal cleanliness and the appearance were considered to be extremely important. Soap was unknown in Egypt but a refreshing body scrub could be made from a mixture of powdered calcite, red natron, salt and honey (Eb 715). Rich and poor washed frequently and before every meal. Much use was made of ointments to keep the skin soft, and unguents and aromatic oils were considered extremely important. At banquets and on other occasions men and women wore lumps of animal fat on top of their wigs or hair (figure 56). These were impregnated with perfume and, as the fat melted, it ran down the body, drenching it with scent. Deodorants were made from ground carob-pod pulp (Eb 709) or a mixture of incense and porridge rolled into pellets (Eb 711).

Women shaved their bodies with bronze razors and used tweezers to pluck out stray hairs. A prescription for a depilatory included the boiled and crushed bones of a bird mixed with fly dung, oil, sycamore juice, gum and cucumber (Hearst Papyrus 155). Men were generally clean-shaven; often the head was also shaved. Herdsmen who guarded the cattle in the pastures were the exception and were often depicted with beards. In a climate where parasites, fleas and lice were plentiful, hair provided a natural and attractive habitat and lice eggs have been found in the hair of mummies.

Although translations of various texts have suggested the symptoms of venereal disease, there is no clear evidence for its existence. However, prostitution was an established aspect of sexual behaviour and, although adultery was officially condemned, there is textual evidence from Deir el-Medina of both adultery and abortions. A man might legitimately have a mistress while he remained unmarried but polygamy and the possession of concubines appear to be rare outside the royal family and high society. The evidence from Deir el-Medina suggests that a woman's legal status regarding marriage, ownership of property and inheritance was equal to that of her husband. Consanguineous marriage was rare except amongst the royal family, where a Pharaoh might marry his sister or daughter in order to establish an inheritance through the female line.

Sexual deviation such as bestiality, necrophilia and homosexuality are not well attested. The Dream Books contain references to the coupling of men and women with certain animals but these dreams were usually considered to be bad omens. Herodotus, writing in the fifth century BC, observed that the beautiful wives of notable men were not delivered to the embalmers until several days after death in order to lessen the chances of violation of their bodies. Lastly, there is the apocryphal tale, written on a Twenty-fifth Dynasty papyrus (Louvre E25351), of the Pharaoh Pepi II (Sixth Dynasty), who enjoyed an illicit relationship with his general, Sisene.

Although age at marriage varied, Egyptian girls usually married at twelve or thirteen and the boys a year or so older, immediately upon reaching sexual maturity. A study of 709 Dynastic skulls from sites at Asyut and Gebelein (housed in the Institute of Anthropology, Turin) revealed the average age at death to be 36 years.

The Egyptians delighted in the birth of a child and probably breast-fed into the subsequent pregnancy (figure 5). Wealthy women employed wet nurses. Prescriptions for galactagogues (substances which increase the flow of milk) may be found in the Ebers Papyrus (Eb 836, 837). However, the likelihood of all live births flourishing to adulthood was small and giving birth brought its own hazards. The hieroglyphs meaning 'to give birth' provide information about the way Egyptian women had their babies (figures 6 and 7). They adopted a squatting position rather than a recumbent one for the actual birth and they used a birthing stool or birthing bricks which raised the body sufficiently above the ground to allow room for the newborn infant. The Westcar Papyrus (*c.*1650-1550 BC) says of the infant: 'They washed it, cut off its navel cord, and laid it on the bed of bricks...'.

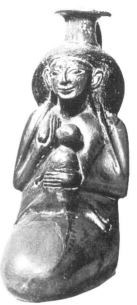

5. Glazed terracotta vase depicting a woman breast-feeding. Such vases were probably intended to hold human milk which was used as a constituent in remedies. (Courtesy of the Musée du Louvre, Paris, AF.1660.)

Studies of mummies have revealed horrific birth injuries which were fatal in some cases and undoubtedly caused chronic disability in others. Princess Hehenhit (Eleventh Dynasty) died soon after giving birth. She had a vesicovaginal fistula which must have caused severe postpartum infection. This distressing condition, commonly a result of poor care in childbirth, was recognised in the Kahun Papyrus:

> Prescription for a woman whose urine is in an irksome place: if the urine keeps coming ... and she distinguishes it, she will be like this forever ... (K 34).

6. The hieroglyphs meaning 'to give birth' depict a squatting position and the use of a birthing stool or birthing bricks. (Drawing by Helena Jaeschke.)

The first successful operation for vesicovaginal fistula was not performed until 1849 by the American gynaecologist James Marion Sims.

Vaginal and rectal prolapse have been found in several specimens although the embalming technique of evisceration through the anus may present a similar pathological appearance. *The Archaeological Survey of Nubia* (1908) mentions a deformed Coptic negress who died in childbirth as a result of a congenitally absent sacro-iliac joint which prevented the pelvis from expanding during labour. An interesting finding by Elliot Smith and Dawson (1924) was of a pregnant sixteen-year-old who was buried unceremoniously after meeting a violent death. They postulated illegitimate conception.

When Petrie was excavating Kahun, he found, buried beneath the earthen floors of some of the houses, boxes which contained the bodies of babies. Infant burials, placed within the precincts of the dwelling, have been found at Predynastic and Dynastic sites, probably to ensure the safe delivery and survival of the next child, or so that the spirit of the dead baby would re-enter the mother's body in a new conception. This practice was recorded in Upper Egypt in the AD 1920s. Although Petrie brought back several of the wooden boxes from Kahun (now in the Manchester Museum and the Petrie Museum of Egyptian Archaeology, University College London), the small bodies can no longer be traced for autopsy.

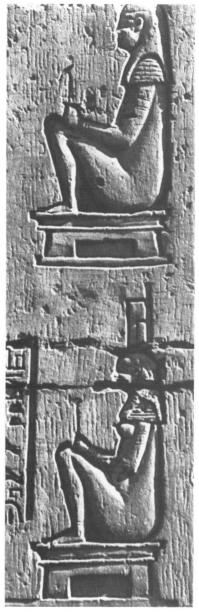

7. (Above right) Wall relief of women seated on birthing stools from the temple, Kom Ombo, Roman Period. (Photograph David G. Burder, FRPS.)

3
The medical profession

In Egypt, as in most early civilisations, men felt secure when they were at peace with the transcendental world and, because religion and magic dominated all aspects of life, both magico-religious and empirico-rational medicine existed side by side.

According to a Christian writer, Alexandrinus Clemens, living in Alexandria in about AD 200, the priests of Early Dynastic Egypt had written the sum total of their knowledge in 42 sacred books kept in the temples and carried in religious processions. Six of these books were concerned totally with medicine and dealt with anatomy, diseases in general, surgery, remedies, diseases of the eye and diseases of women. No examples of these books survive nor of the anatomy books said to have been written by Athothis, second Pharaoh of the First Dynasty.

During the Old Kingdom the medical profession became highly organised, with doctors holding a variety of ranks and specialities. The ordinary doctor or *sinw* was outranked by the *imy-r sinw* (overseer of doctors) the *wr sinw* (chief of doctors), the *smsw sinw* (eldest of doctors) and the *shd sinw* (inspector of doctors). Above all these practitioners was the overseer of doctors of Upper and Lower Egypt. There is evidence that a distinction was made between physicians and surgeons, the latter being known as the 'priests of the goddess Sekhmet'. There were also healers who used purely magical remedies or exorcism.

The hieroglyphs for *sinw* were usually written showing the man, the pot of medicine and the lancet. Sometimes this was written with the determinative sign showing an old man leaning on a stick. This was the hieroglyphic epithet for 'old age' and probably indicated that the physician in question was a venerable doctor of many years standing (figure 8).

From the whole of the Pharaonic era, the names and titles of about a hundred doctors are known with sufficient detail to uncover an overall picture of medical practice. The name of Imhotep has become inextricably linked with Egyptian medicine (figure 9). He was vizier, architect and chief physician to the Pharaoh Djoser (Third Dynasty) and during the Greek Period he was deified and identified with Asklepios, the Greek god of healing.

Hesire, a contemporary of Imhotep, was chief of physicians and also a dentist (figure 10). The practice of dentistry in ancient Egypt is much disputed. Certainly, as has been noted, dental disease was very common. The discovery, in a Fourth Dynasty grave at Giza, of several teeth wired together has suggested to some that a dental conservationist at-

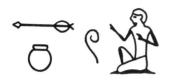

8. The word for *sinw* or 'physician' was written showing the man, the pot of medicine and the lancet. (Drawing by Helena Jaeschke.)

tempted to manufacture a dental bridge.

Iry was chief of court physicians at Giza during the Fourth Dynasty. He was also 'master of scorpions', 'eye doctor of the palace', 'doctor of the abdomen' and 'guardian of the royal bowel movement' (figure 11). Sekhet-n-Ankh was 'nose doctor' to Pharaoh Sahure (Fifth Dynasty) and successfully cured him of a 'sickness of the upper air passages'.

The only Egyptian lady doctor yet known was Peseshet (Fourth or early Fifth Dynasty), whose title, *imy-rt-swnt*, may be translated as 'lady director of lady physicians'.

Each specialisation of medicine had a patron god or goddess and the physician worked directly under the auspices of his particular deity. Duaw was the god of eye diseases; Taurt was a goddess of childbirth, as was Hathor. Sekhmet, the lion-headed lady of pestilence, sent plagues all over the land and Horus had power over deadly stings and bites such as those of crocodiles, snakes and scorpions (the most common type of 'everyday' injury appears to have been from bites). The human body was divided into 36 parts and each part came under the protection of a god or goddess. The goddess protecting the liver was Isis; that of the lungs was Nephthys; the stomach was the domain of Neith and the intestines belonged to the care of Selket.

The House of Life (Per Ankh)

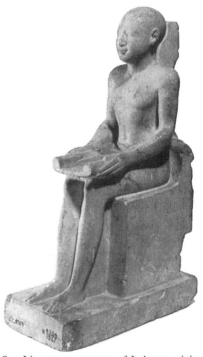

9. Limestone statuette of Imhotep, vizier and chief physician to Pharaoh Djoser. (Courtesy of the Petrie Museum of Egyptian Archaeology, University College London, UC 8709.)

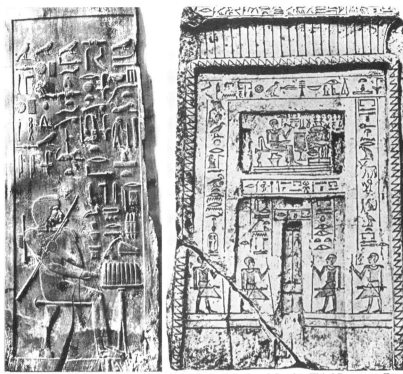

10. (Left) Wood relief of Hesire, a chief of physicians and dentist, Third Dynasty. From the mastaba of Hesire, Saqqara. (Courtesy of the Egyptian Museum, Cairo, JE 28504.)

11. (Right) Limestone stele of Iry, a chief of court physicians, Fourth Dynasty. Amongst other specialities, Iry was 'guardian of the royal bowel movement'. (From Junker, *H. Der Hofarzt Irj. Zeitschrift für ägyptische Sprache*, 1928: 63.)

was the medical study centre where doctors were taught and these existed at major cult temples along with centres of healing. The remains of the magnificent temple excavated at Edfu date from the Greek Period although the western side has an inner and an outer enclosure which date to the Old Kingdom (figure 12). There was a herb garden to the right of the building in which many of the ingredients for the physicians' remedies and prescriptions would have been grown.

The temples at Dendera, Deir el-Bahri and Philae were also used for therapeutic purposes during the Greek and Roman Periods. At Dendera there was a sacred lake and mudbrick sanatorium where visitors were anointed with water which had first been poured over healing statues, or they could spend the night in the hope of being healed by the goddess

Hathor. At Deir el-Bahri the upper terrace was consecrated to Imhotep and a special room was built for his worship. Numerous graffiti are evidence of the large number of invalids who visited it until the second century AD. Most of them are dedicated to Asklepios, often associated with his daughter, Hygieia.

Sick people seeking help at the temples were expected to make an offering to the gods (figure 13). This provided a useful source of income for the temple. Offerings were made according to means — perhaps cloth, bread, fruit, or, from wealthier patients, an ox or jewellery. Some patients underwent 'sleep therapy', whereby a twilight sleep was induced by administering opium or an extract of the mandrake, and the sick person's demons were thus exorcised. Possibly, too, other more painful treatments may have been carried out whilst the patient was semi-conscious. Very often the sick person left a model of the area of the body which contained his pain or sickness so that the

12. Reconstruction of the temple at Edfu, Greek Period. Some of the herbs from the herb garden to the right of the temple would have been used for making medicines. (Courtesy of the Bettmann Archive.)

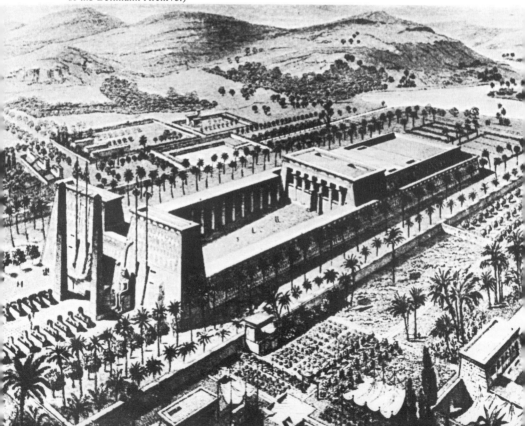

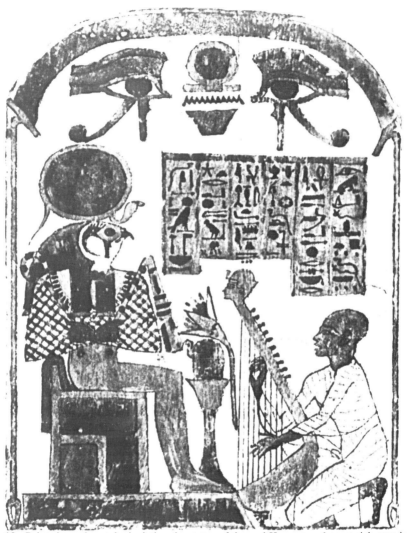

13. Painted wooden stele depicting the statue of the god Horus, to whom a sick man is bringing gifts, Third Intermediate Period. (Courtesy of the Musée du Louvre, Paris, N 3657.)

temple medicine might go on working while he remained outside its precincts. Amulets were worn to ward off sickness and tiny protective statuettes were kept in many homes.

Large collections of medical writings were kept in the temples even as late as the second century AD, when Galen wrote that Greek physicians still visited the library of the school at Memphis.

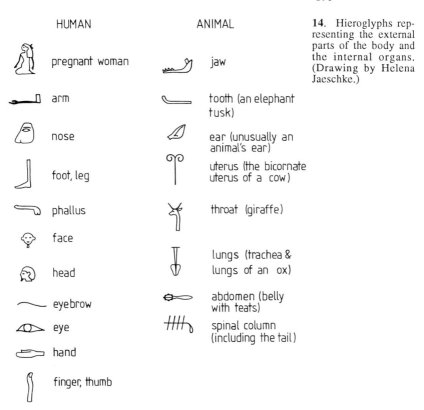

HUMAN

pregnant woman

arm

nose

foot, leg

phallus

face

head

eyebrow

eye

hand

finger, thumb

ANIMAL

jaw

tooth (an elephant tusk)

ear (unusually an animal's ear)

uterus (the bicornate uterus of a cow)

throat (giraffe)

lungs (trachea & lungs of an ox)

abdomen (belly with teats)

spinal column (including the tail)

14. Hieroglyphs representing the external parts of the body and the internal organs. (Drawing by Helena Jaeschke.)

The hieroglyphic signs for the external parts of the body are mostly derived from human anatomy whilst the signs for internal organs are derived from animal parts (figure 14). Whilst this provides some evidence to suggest that the Egyptians did not dissect human bodies, descriptions of injuries from the Old Kingdom text of the Edwin Smith Papyrus suggest otherwise. A vertebral crush injury causing tetraplegia is so accurately described that anatomical exposure of the cervical spine may have been performed.

Although no surgical scars have been reported in mummies (apart from embalmers' incisions), there are thirteen references in the Smith Papyrus to *ydr*, which the Egyptologist James Breasted translated as 'stitching'. The papyrus also mentions wounds being brought together with adhesive tape which was made of linen. Linen was also available for bandages, ligatures and sutures. Needles were probably of copper.

A box of surgical instruments was carved in relief on the outer corridor wall of the temple at Kom Ombo, which dates from the Roman

Period (figure 15). These include metal shears, surgical knives and saws, probes and spatulas, small hooks and forceps. An oculist's box of instruments, as well as surgical instruments resembling cauteries and scalpels (Late Period), has also been found.

Egyptian doctors distinguished between sterile (clean) wounds and infected (purulent) wounds. The former were written using the determinative for 'blood' or 'phlegm' and the latter using the determinative for 'stinking outflow' or 'faeces' (figure 16). A mixture of ibex fat, fir oil and crushed peas was used in an ointment to clean an infected wound (Eb 522b).

Sometimes the hieroglyphs provide insight into disease analogy and symptom recognition. The word for 'sweat' was written using the pictogram determinative for 'water' and the word for 'inflammation' used the

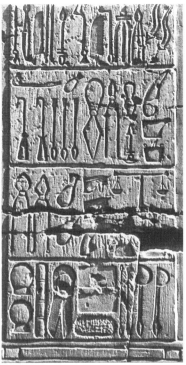

15. (Above) Wall relief of surgical instruments from the temple, Kom Ombo, Roman Period. (Photograph David G. Burder, FRPS.)

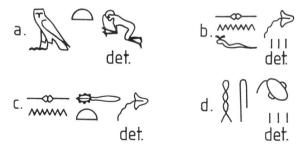

16. Words using the 'outpouring' determinatives. (a) A disease for which no cure could be found or an unnaturally occurring illness such as an accident. (b) Blood — where fluid issues from the lips. (c) Phlegm — using the same determinative as (b). (d) Faeces — where the determinative means 'stinking outflow'. (Drawing by Helena Jaeschke.)

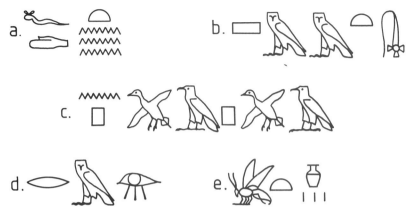

17. The words for (a) 'sweat', (b) 'inflammation', (c) 'flutter', (d) 'weep' and (e) 'honey'. (Drawing by Helena Jaeschke.)

sign for a brazier. The word for 'flutter' was written using pictograms representing fluttering birds. Similar pictorial representations are used to convey the meaning of the words 'weep' and 'honey' (figure 17). The word for 'injury', also meaning 'to smite', shows a man about to strike an assailant with a stick (figure 18a). An illness causing shortness of breath would be written using the determinative of a 'sail' (figure 18b). Putting a fractured or dislocated bone back into its place was represented by two crossed bones (figure 18c).

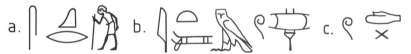

18. The hieroglyphs are often synonymous with the nature of an ailment, hence the words for a disease caused by (a) injury, (b) breathlessness and (c) a fractured or dislocated bone. (Drawing by Helena Jaeschke.)

A plaster for setting a fracture might be made from cow's milk mixed with barley (Hearst Papyrus 219) or acacia leaves (*Acacia nilotica* Desf.) mixed with gum and water (Hearst Papyrus 223). Two Fifth Dynasty fractures had been set with bark splints and bandages. Bandages and poultices were used to apply therapeutic substances to lesions and to 'draw out' poisons from internal ailments. A poultice of porridge and myrtle (*Myrtus communis* L.) was used to 'remove mucus' from the right or left side of the chest (Berlin Papyrus 142) — perhaps this was lobar pneumonia or pleurisy. The binding bases of other poultices were clay, sawdust, wax and pondweed.

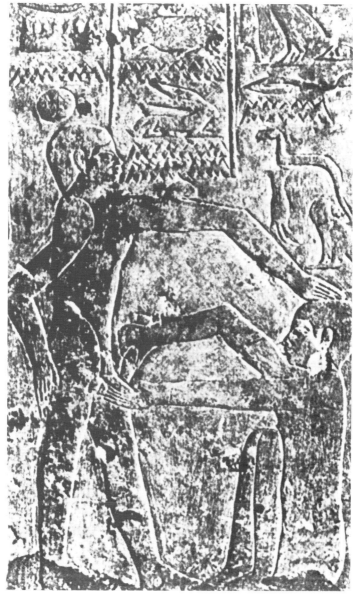

19. Wall relief depicting a circumcision scene. From the mastaba of Ankh-ma-Hor, Saqqara, Sixth Dynasty. (From A. P. Leca, *La Médecine Égyptienne au Temps des Pharaons*, Roger Dacosta, Paris, 1983. Plate XVI.)

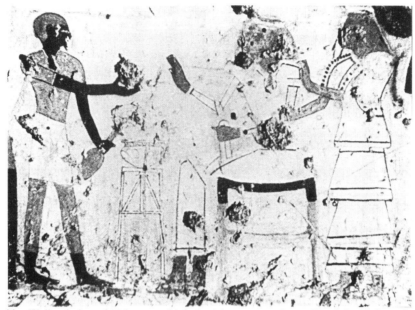

20. Wall painting of Nebamun, chief physician to Amenhotep II, of the Eighteenth Dynasty, giving a remedy to a prince of Mesopotamia who has requested medical aid. (From Walter Wreszinski, *Atlas zur altägyptischen Kulturgeschichte*, Leipzig 1923, t.I, pl.115.)

A wall relief from the tomb of Ankh-ma-Hor at Saqqara depicts a circumcision scene (figure 19). There seems to be no reason why some Pharaohs, priests and officials were circumcised and others were not. The Greek historian Strabo claimed that the Egyptians also practised female circumcision but examinations of female mummies show that they have either not been circumcised or their condition is too decayed to be able to tell.

From the New Kingdom onwards Egyptian doctors were to be found as advisors or chief physicians at many of the most important foreign courts, notably in Anatolia, Syria, Persia and Mesopotamia (figure 20). Expeditionary forces posted to Punt, Crete and Phoenicia were also equipped with doctors. The Greek historian Diodorus Siculus wrote:

> In wartime, and on journeys anywhere within Egypt, the phys-
> icians draw their support from public funds and administer their
> treatments in accordance with a written law which was composed
> in ancient times by many famous physicians.

A Middle Kingdom mass grave (*c*.2000 BC) held the bodies of sixty soldiers who had fought in the north to reunite the country. Their wounds included arrow holes (with arrows *in situ*) and bludgeonings. A general who fought an elephant during the reign of Tuthmosis III (Eighteenth Dynasty) sustained a superficial scalp wound.

Herodotus says that it was an Egyptian oculist who aided the Persian Cambyses, son of Cyrus the Great, in his invasion of Egypt when he founded the Twenty-seventh Dynasty in 525 BC. The treacherous doctor was seeking revenge on the Pharaoh Ahmose II for sending him from his family to the Persian court.

By the time of the Persian invasion, it appears that medicine had suffered from the growing internal troubles and threats of invasion prevalent in the Late Period. User-hor-Resinet was chief of physicians to Darius I (521-486 BC), who, it appears, was concerned about this decline in medical practice:

His Majesty, Darius I, lord of all lands and of Egypt also ... ordered me to go to Sais in Egypt. He instructed me to restore the 'houses of life' which had fallen into disrepair. I did as His Majesty commanded ... I filled them with students from the families of the nobles — taking no sons of the poor. I placed them in charge of wise men ... His Majesty commanded me to provide them with all that they needed, with all instruments, according to the drawings of the old times ....

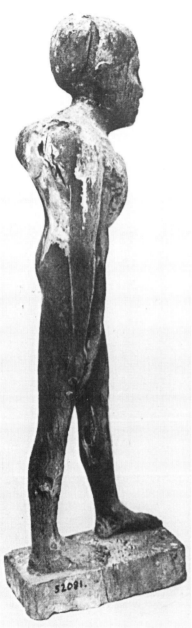

21. (Left) Wooden figurine depicting kyphosis of the spine and concomitant deformity of the chest. These may be due to Pott's disease but are more likely to be a congenital deformity, Fifth Dynasty. (Courtesy of the Egyptian Museum, Cairo, JE 52081.)

22. (Below) Red clay statuette from Aswan depicting Pott's disease — tuberculous osteomyelitis of the spine, Predynastic. (Private collection, Paris.)

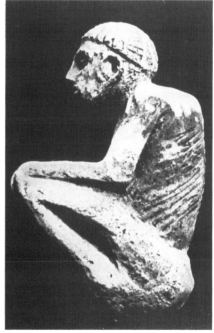

4
Diseases and deformities

Although literary evidence suggests that leprosy was established in China during the first millennium BC, its introduction into Egypt may have come via the armies of Alexander the Great returning from India in 327-326 BC. Certainly the earliest skeletal evidence of leprosy is from the Dakhleh Oasis in Egypt. A Greek Period cemetery contained the skeletons of four adult males of European type who were diagnosed by Dzierzykray-Rogalski in 1980. It has been suggested that these Europeans, in a predominantly negroid burial ground, represented lepers banished from the Ptolemaic capital of Alexandria because of their disease. Only two further acceptable cases of leprosy have been discovered in Egypt. These Coptic Christian bodies date from the fourth century AD and were found in a cemetery at el-Bigha, Nubia, and examined by Elliot Smith and Derry in 1910. They have been extensively re-examined since the 1960s by Rowling, Møller-Christensen and Sandison.

The bacteria causing leprosy (*Mycobacterium leprae*) and those causing tuberculosis (*Mycobacterium tuberculosis*) are of the same genus and the earliest evidence of human tuberculosis is from Egypt, where, unlike leprosy, it was a relatively common disease. It is likely that man obtained his first tuberculosis bacillus from the close contact with livestock (bovine tuberculosis) which occurred after the neolithic revolution. Although the infection largely affects soft tissue, bone involvement occurs in 5-7 per cent of cases of untreated tuberculosis. Figurines demonstrating the angular kyphosis characteristic of Pott's tuberculous osteomyelitis of the spine may date from before 3000 BC (figures 21 and 22). The mummy of the Twenty-first Dynasty priest Nesperehan has been accepted as a typical case of Pott's disease with characteristic abscess in the psoas muscle. Evidence for pulmonary tuberculosis is less tenable because the bacilli disappear soon after the death of their victim. The discovery of fibrous adhesions and pneumothorax in mummies has been cited as evidence for its existence but other respiratory conditions may cause these pathological changes.

In 1910 Margaret Murray found evidence of sand pneumoconiosis in a male mummy and this is now known to have been a fairly common condition in ancient Egypt. As part of the Manchester Museum Mummy Project which began in the 1970s, several specimens have undergone endoscopic examination. A rigid industrial endoscope was used to visualise the inside of the thorax of a male mummy called Khary. Khary's pulmonary adhesions caused by sand pneumoconiosis were so

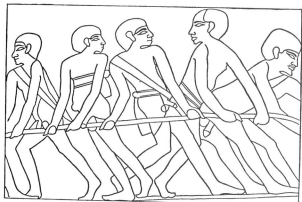

23. Five fishermen show evidence of schistosomiasis — umbilical herniae, enlarged scrotal sacs and gynaecomastia. The man on the far right has generalised genital hypertrophy. From the tomb of Mehu, Sixth Dynasty, Saqqara.

severe that they divided the chest cavity into three sections. The lungs of the mummy known as PUM II (Philadelphia University Museum), unwrapped in Detroit in 1973, contained a silica content of 0.22 per cent (the normal is 0.05 per cent or less). Another common finding in Egyptian remains is anthracosis, attributable to environmental pollution from cooking and burning fires and oil lamps in small rooms.

In 1910 the palaeopathologist Sir Marc Armand Ruffer found the calcified eggs of the Bilharzia worm (*Schistosoma haematobium* or *Schistosoma mansoni*) in the preserved kidneys of two mummies of the Twentieth Dynasty. This worm develops in the viscera of a species of snail which resides in the mud of the Nile's irrigation canals, enters the human body chiefly through the skin and takes up residence in the kidney, bladder and intestines. Schistosomiasis victims suffer cirrhosis of the liver, retention of abdominal fluid (ascites), chronic exhaustion, bloody urine (haematuria — mentioned about fifty times in the medical literature) and often fatal haemorrhages. Visible manifestations of the infestation include breast enlargement (noted specifically in the male and termed 'gynaecomastia'), secondary to liver cirrhosis, and enlarged scrotal sacs and umbilical hernias due to the increase in abdominal pressure resulting from ascites. The mummy of Ramesses V reveals an enlarged, eviscerated scrotal sac.

There are wall reliefs in two Old Kingdom tombs at Saqqara in which various body swellings, indicative of schistosomiasis, are depicted. In one illustration there is a small umbilical protrusion on a man carrying bundles of papyrus and in another a jousting sailor has a similar protrusion. A grain cutter has an umbilical hernia and an enlarged scrotal sac whilst the five men in yet another illustration show evidence of these last two, as well as genital hypertrophy and gynaecomastia (figure 23). A potter has gross genital hypertrophy (figure 24).

24. Wall relief of a potter with gross genital hypertrophy. From the tomb of Mehou, Sixth Dynasty, Saqqara.

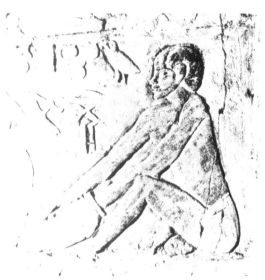

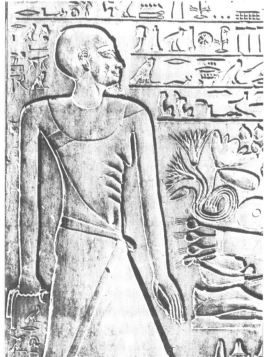

25. Limestone wall relief of a male showing the pendulous breasts of old age, Twelfth Dynasty. (Courtesy of the Musée du Louvre, Paris, C 2.)

The gynaecomastia of schistosomiasis must not be confused with the large breasts depicted in elderly men which denoted veneration in achieving the wisdom of old age. Here the breasts were always shown as pendulous (figure 25).

The microscopic *Schistosoma haematobium* was discovered only in 1851 (by Theodor Bilharz) but the Egyptians had plenty of other very visible worms to worry about: *Strongyloides*, Guinea worm, *Taenia*, *Ascaris* and *Trichinella* were all very common and three cases merit attention.

A lung biopsy was obtained endoscopically from a female mummy called Asru in the Manchester Museum. Histology revealed part of the wall of a hydatid cyst which in life might have measured 20 cm in diameter and made Asru breathless with a chronic cough. Hydatid disease is caused by the larval stage of the dog tapeworm *Echinococcus granulosus*. Infection occurs when infested food is eaten and cysts may develop in many organs, including the brain. Within the skull, which cannot expand to accommodate a growing mass, the cyst becomes a 'space-occupying lesion' and often proves fatal. This is almost certainly how Manchester mummy 22940 met his death, for attached to his brain cyst were the heads of developing tapeworms.

The mummy of a weaver named Nakht from the court of Pharaoh Sethnakhte (Twentieth Dynasty) was examined at Toronto University in 1974. Nakht was between fourteen and eighteen years old and infested with *Taenia*, *Trichinella spiralis* and *Schistosoma haematobium*. He had evidence of early liver cirrhosis and congestive splenomegaly (the spleen had ruptured). Red blood cells found in the bladder suggested haematuria in life. Infestation by the parasite *Trichinella spiralis* occurs through eating inadequately cooked pork.

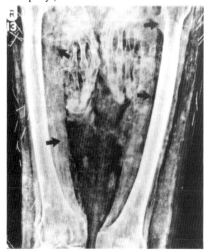

26. X-ray of the legs of a mummy (Twenty-first Dynasty) showing calcification of the femoral arteries (arrows) seen in arteriosclerosis. (Courtesy of the Eastman Kodak Company.)

The pathogenesis of vascular disease has only in recent years become clarified but arterial degenerative disease (arteriosclerosis) was not uncommon in Egypt and has been found to a considerable degree in mummies of Egyptians who died very young (figure 26).

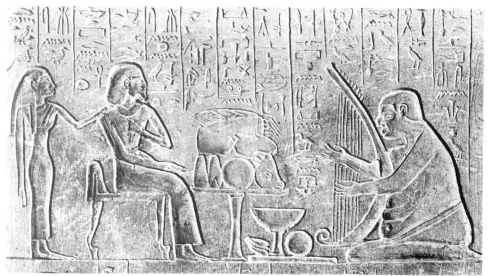

27. Wall relief of Neferhotep, a grossly obese harpist, playing before the prince Aki, Middle Kingdom. (Courtesy of the Rijksmuseum van Oudheden, Leiden, AP 25.)

The Pharaoh Ramesses II lived until he was over ninety but Elliot Smith (1912) observed tortuous, calcified temporal arteries in the head of his mummy and extreme calcareous degeneration of the aorta in his younger but still mature son, Merneptah. Ruffer described arteriosclerosis in mummies from the New Kingdom to the Greek and Coptic Periods. The mummy of Lady Teye (Twenty-first Dynasty), aged about fifty, who lived at Deir el-Bahri, showed evidence of atheromatous disease of the aorta with calcification of the coronary artery and mitral valve. She also had arteriosclerosis of the kidney, which would have contributed to a serious rise in blood pressure.

Arteriosclerosis is sometimes associated with obesity and studies of the skin folds of mummies such as those of the Pharaohs Amenophis III and Ramesses III showed that they were immensely fat, although obesity was generally not depicted in their portraits for reasons of etiquette (figure 27). Obesity may also be associated with inflammation of the gall bladder (cholecystitis) and gall-stone formation (cholelithiasis). Pathological and radiological evidence of gall-stones has been found in several mummies, notably females, in whom they are most common (figure 28).

A rather unusual depiction of obesity appears on a wall painting in the temple of Queen Hatshepsut at Deir el-Bahri, where an epic voyage to the land of Punt (modern Somalia) was recorded. The Queen of Punt's deformities have been generally diagnosed as Dercum's disease (neuro-

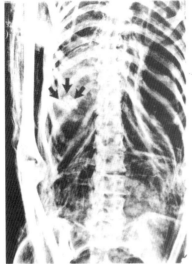

lipomatosis dolorosa), a disorder largely restricted to females which produces nerve lesions and localised painful accumulations of subcutaneous fat (figure 29). It is not unlikely, however, that the queen was simply overweight. Later Meroitic queens (Graeco-Roman Period) were represented in similar style, and in recent centuries the wealth and status of certain African tribal leaders was emphasised by the size of their wives. The original wall painting included the queen's two sons and a daughter, who was becoming obese.

28. (Above) X-ray of a female mummy showing a cluster of gall-stones in the gall bladder (arrows). Gall-stones may often be associated with obesity and diet. (Courtesy of the Eastman Kodak Company.)

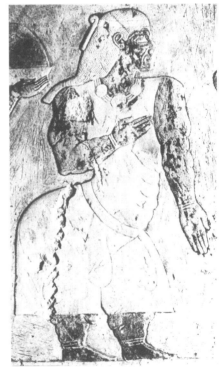

29. (Right) Painted wall relief of the Queen of Punt with deformities suggestive of Dercum's disease. From the temple of Queen Hatshepsut, Deir el-Bahri, Eighteenth Dynasty. (Courtesy of the Egyptian Museum, Cairo, TR-12-11-26-5 [temporary number].)

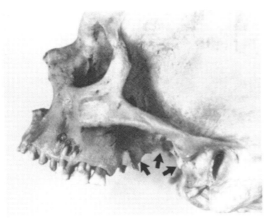

30. (Left) Multiple basal-cell naevus syndrome showing cavitation (arrows) of left maxilla in relation to the first molar. This large cystic cavity may have become secondarily infected following the pulpal exposure. Male aged sixty to seventy years, excavated at Asyut. (Courtesy of the Institute of Anthropology, University of Turin, E.235.)

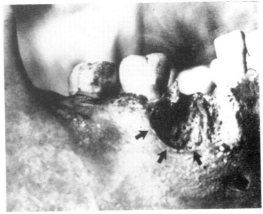

31. (Right) Multiple basal-cell naevus syndrome showing cyst (arrows) in mandible near the right first molar, which had been shed during life. This was probably a dentigerous (tooth-containing) cyst. Male aged twenty to twenty-five years, excavated at Asyut. (Courtesy of the Institute of Anthropology, University of Turin, E.225.)

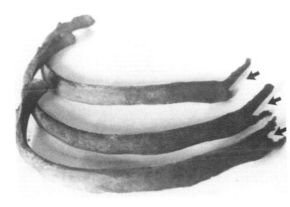

32. (Left) Multiple basal-cell naevus syndrome showing three bifid ribs (arrows) which are broadened anteriorly and posteriorly. From same skeleton as figure 30. (Courtesy of the Institute of Anthropology, University of Turin, E.235.)

Although the medical papyri deal with various disorders of the alimentary tract, little has been written about alimentary diseases in mummies. Elliot Smith and Wood Jones (1910) described gross appendicular adhesions, which probably followed appendicitis, in a Byzantine body. Rectal prolapse and infantile megacolon (Hirschsprung's disease) have been found in mummies of the Roman Period.

Skin which has undergone adequate dehydration before mummification and which has not been badly damaged by the embalming process retains much of its lifelike appearance. Skin diseases such as solar keratosis, keratosis senilis, ulcers and malignant squamous papilloma have been recognised in several mummies. It is almost certain that Ramesses V did not die from his scrotal hernia but from smallpox. His perfectly preserved head is covered with the distinctive pustules of this virulent infection.

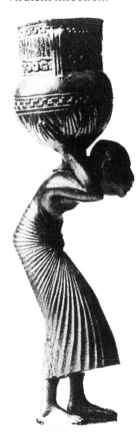

A rare condition, which in life would be recognised by its dermatological appearance but in death was diagnosed by its associated skeletal abnormalities, is multiple basal-cell naevus syndrome. This genetic abnormality, first described in 1960, presents with hundreds of naevi and malignant nodules covering the face and trunk. There are associated cystic lesions of the jaw, bifid ribs, scoliosis, polydactyly (extra fingers and toes) and facial asymmetry. Two male skeletons, excavated at Asyut, examined in 1967 and now housed in the University of Turin, were found to have this syndrome (figures 30, 31 and 32). Discovered in the same vicinity, they were almost certainly related.

Other more common but equally painful inflammatory and degenerative bone diseases would have had serious consequences for many Egyptians. Arthritis, periostitis and osteomyelitis have been found in an extraordinarily large number of mummies (figures 33 and 34) from Predynastic to Coptic times. Of eight bodies of the New Kingdom and Roman Period

33. Wooden statue of a servant carrying a water jar, Eighteenth Dynasty. His posture, if frequently adopted, might predispose to osteo-arthritis (see figure 34). (Courtesy of the Board of Trustees of the National Museums and Galleries on Merseyside, Liverpool Museum, M 3519.)

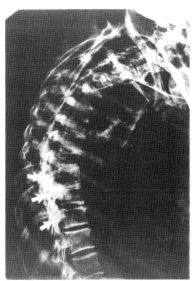

34. X-ray of a mummy showing degenerative changes of the thoracic vertebrae (arrows). (Courtesy of the Field Museum of Natural History, Chicago, neg. no. 74522.)

(housed in the British Museum) which were examined radiologically in 1961, osteoarthritic lipping of the vertebrae was noted in four. Periosteal inflammation may be related to infection or trauma (notably fractures) and is seen particularly on the tibia, which has a large subcutaneous area. In one study of 6000 skeletons, it was found that, although only 3 per cent of Egyptians had ever sustained a fracture, periostitis was not uncommon. This suggests that infection from insect bites or simple abrasions may have been responsible.

The condition of tibial bones also provides a clue to the general state of Egyptian health. Subjected to radiological examination, 30 per cent of 133 mummies screened by Gray during the 1960s show lines of arrested growth (Harris's lines). These indicate episodes of intermittent disease or malnutrition and suggest a generally poor state of health during childhood and adolescence. A study of 185 adult Nubian skeletons revealed significantly higher rates of arrested growth and bone loss (osteoporosis) in females than males. In present-day societies osteoporosis is associated with the ageing process but the Nubian data show an earlier age of onset and a more rapid rate of bone loss. The problems that these young females experienced in bone maintenance were most likely due to the combination of nutritional and reproductive stress.

An osteoporotic fracture of the neck of the femur occurred in an elderly priestess named Nesi-Tet-Nab-Taris (Twenty-first Dynasty). Because of her subsequent immobility, this unfortunate lady developed extensive pressure sores on her buttocks and back. After her death the embalmers attempted to restore the defects by grafting patches of gazelle skin over the raw areas.

No skeletal evidence of the childhood disease of rickets (caused by a deficiency of vitamin D) has been discovered although this could be seen in Egypt in relatively recent times. The intense Egyptian sunlight (which converts natural subcutaneous fats into vitamin D) may have provided some immunity.

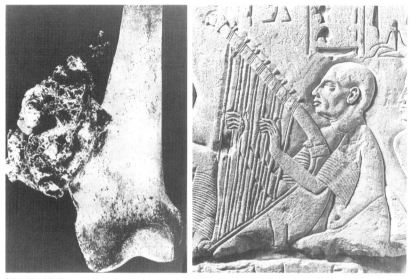

35. (Left) Femur showing a large osteochondroma, Fifth Dynasty. Reproduced from 'Pathological Changes in Mummies', *Proceedings of the Royal Society of Medicine*, volume 54, May 1961, 409-15. (Courtesy of the Royal Society of Medicine and Mr John Thompson Rowling.)

36. (Right) Wall relief of a blind harpist, Eighteenth Dynasty. From the tomb of Paatenhemheb. (Courtesy of the Rijksmuseum van Oudheden, Leiden, AMT 1-35.)

The evidence of malignant tumours in Egyptian remains is largely confined to bone and even these are rare. Malignancies become more common with age, and life expectancy in Egypt was short. Primary carcinomas sometimes cause bone destruction as in the case of sacral erosion due to a possible rectal carcinoma in a Byzantine body and nasal carcinoma in a pre-Christian Nubian. Two skulls of the First and Twentieth Dynasties display evidence of bone changes commonly associated with intracranial meningioma. A diagnostic error occurred in 1924 when a Fifth Dynasty femur illustrated by Elliot Smith and Dawson became labelled 'osteosarcoma' (figure 35). This tumour looks formidable but is a benign osteocartilaginous exostosis or osteochondroma. There are no

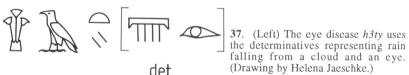

det.

37. (Left) The eye disease *h3ty* uses the determinatives representing rain falling from a cloud and an eye. (Drawing by Helena Jaeschke.)

examples of breast cancer in mummies although the female mummy called PUM III, who died about 835 BC at the age of 35 and was autopsied in Detroit in the 1970s, revealed evidence of a small benign fibroadenoma of the left breast.

A blind musician is depicted in a wall relief from a tomb in the Eighteenth Dynasty (figure 36) and, from another tomb of about the same era, a small group of blind singers kneel to praise the Pharaoh Akhenaten. These entertainers may have been blind from birth but it is quite likely that they contracted one of the many eye diseases prevalent along the banks of the Nile — leucoma, cataract (referred to as 'barleycorn'), conjunctivitis and trachoma (caused by *Chlamydia trachomatis* infection and still known as 'Egyptian eye disease', figure 37).

As well as acquired diseases, undoubtedly a number of Egyptians suffered from inherited and congenital deformities. The dwarfism known as achondroplasia is probably the most frequently depicted of these and is a short-limbed disorder due to a dominant genetic mutation (figures 38 and 39).

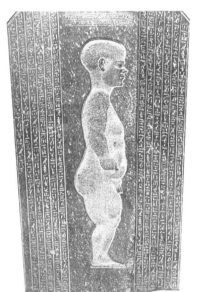 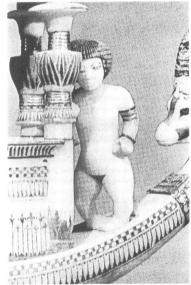

38. (Left) The grey granite lid of a dancer's sarcophagus showing the achondroplasic dwarf Djehor, Late Period. Perhaps he was also an entertainer. (Courtesy of the Egyptian Museum, Cairo. Photograph by the author, JE 47398.)

39. (Right) An ornamental alabaster boat from the tomb of Tutankhamun showing an achondroplasic dwarf at the helm, Eighteenth Dynasty. (Courtesy of the Egyptian Museum, Cairo, JE 62120.)

No Egyptian medical text mentions dwarfism but three words designate short stature — *nmw*, *hw* and *dng*. The word *nmw* is often accompanied by the picture of a small man with a long trunk, short limbs and prominent buttocks. The word *hw* usually denotes shortness and physical insufficiency. The word *dng* is similarly associated with the image of a man with short limbs but it may have meant specifically a 'pygmy'. This word occurs in a letter sent by the young Pharaoh Pepi II (Sixth Dynasty) to Harkhuf, the governor of Upper Egypt. Harkhuf had led an expedition to the southern country of Yam in the Sudan and had brought back a small man from the land of Akhtiu at the south-eastern limits of the known world.

The pictorial representation of dwarfs became stereotyped very early and Predynastic examples of small ivory figures have been found at Ballas and Naqada in Upper Egypt. These represent male and female short-limbed dwarfs standing naked with shaven heads and large protuberant ears, short arms and small, bowed legs. More than fifty Old Kingdom tombs, most of them at Giza and Saqqara, bear pictures of short people tending animals, carrying toilet objects or making jewellery. Sitting dwarfs often have peculiar irregularities like spinal humps which could represent kyphosis, a relatively frequent spinal deformity.

Seneb, shown seated with his wife and their normal-limbed children, was an important Sixth Dynasty palace official (figure 40). His several positions included 'overseer of weaving in the palace', 'leader of the administration of the crown of Lower Egypt' and 'leader of the Dwarfs of the Wardrobe'. Seneb has normal facial features and on the false door of his monument the artist reproduced the bodily disproportion of Seneb but followed the standard artistic convention by making him as tall as his servants and even sometimes slightly taller, in order to indicate his superior social status.

Ptah-Sokar, the patron god of craftsmen, known from the Old Kingdom, is depicted in amulets as a dwarf with a flat skullcap or skull. Figures of dwarf demons, called Bes as a generic name, became very popular in the New

40. Painted limestone statue of the dwarf Seneb with his wife, Senetites, and normal-limbed children, Sixth Dynasty. (Courtesy of the Egyptian Museum, Cairo, JE 51280.)

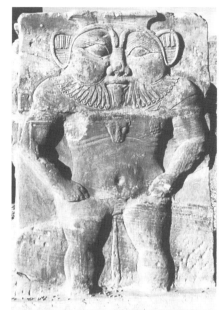

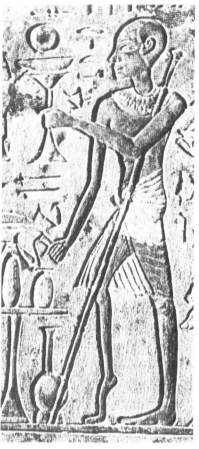

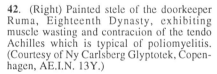

41. (Above) Limestone statue of a Bes-god depicted as a dwarf, Graeco-Roman Period, Dendera. (Photograph David G. Burder, FRPS.)

42. (Right) Painted stele of the doorkeeper Ruma, Eighteenth Dynasty, exhibiting muscle wasting and contraction of the tendo Achilles which is typical of poliomyelitis. (Courtesy of Ny Carlsberg Glyptotek, Copenhagen, AE.I.N. 13Y.)

Kingdom and Later Period as familiar protectors of women in labour and children. Bes-gods have large heads, long trunks and bandy legs (figure 41). For some scholars they resemble cretinous dwarfs but their hybridisation of human and animal features was probably stylistic.

Other congenital conditions observed in mummies include hydrocephalus, cleft palate, hip-joint dysplasia and talipes equinovarus (club foot). This last condition has been the cause of differential diagnosis in several individuals, namely Khnum-Nakht (Twelfth Dynasty) and the Pharaoh Siptah (Nineteenth Dynasty). Early authorities held that both deformities were likely to have been caused by poliomyelitis. Later experts tend to opt for talipes equinovarus. An interesting wall painting from the Eighteenth Dynasty depicts a poor doorkeeper named Ruma

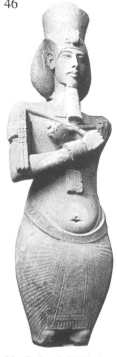

who is making offerings to the goddess Ishtar to cure him of a crippling disease (figure 42). Ruma's wasted right leg and contracted tendo Achilles are characteristic of post-infective poliomyelitis.

The most vehemently argued medical history of the Egyptian period is that of the Pharaoh Akhenaten and his family. Akhenaten, the tenth Pharaoh of the Eighteenth Dynasty, ascended the throne as Amenophis IV. Changing his name, he swept aside the pantheon of gods under the priesthood of Amun and decreed that the royal court would worship only the solar disc — the sun-god Aten. He moved the royal capital from Thebes to a site known as Tell el-Amarna and named his new city Akhetaten — 'the horizon of Aten'.

Statues and paintings reveal Akhenaten's physique to be effeminate with gynaecomastia, swollen

43. (Left) Sandstone statue of Akhenaten revealing his effeminate physique. From the Temple of Aten, Karnak, Eighteenth Dynasty. (Courtesy of the Egyptian Museum, Cairo. Photograph: David G. Burder, FRPS, JE 49529.)

44. (Below left) Black granite statue of Tuthmosis IV, grandfather of Akhenaten, revealing pronounced gynaecomastia. Eighteenth Dynasty. (Courtesy of the Egyptian Museum, Cairo, JE 36336.)

45. (Below right) Sandstone stele of Amenophis III, Akhenaten's father. Amenophis III is shown with gynaecomastia and is dressed in effeminate attire. It must be emphasised that this period produced artistic trends towards femininity. Poses were more relaxed, informal and naturalistic. Eighteenth Dynasty. (Courtesy of the Trustees of the British Museum, London, 57399.)

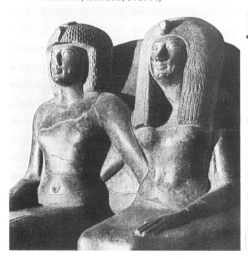

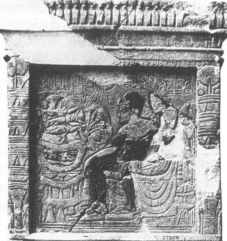

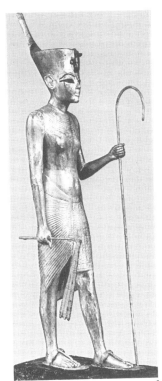

46. Gilded wooden statuette of Tutankhamun showing his gynaecomastia, Eighteenth Dynasty. (Courtesy of the Egyptian Museum, Cairo, JE 60712.)

hips and slightly protuberant abdomen (figure 43). His elongated head, prominent chin and fleshy lips portray an altogether sensuous face. In the absence of Akhenaten's mummy, the diagnoses made on the paintings and statues have been many and varied. Suggestions include a tumour of the pituitary gland causing hormonal imbalance with consequent overgrowth and thickening of bone (acromegaly) and familial incomplete pseudohermaphroditism, a complex feminisation syndrome which is passed through female carriers to their male progeny. Men with severe manifestations of this condition are invariably infertile but, married to the legendary Nefertiti, Akhenaten produced six daughters. However, incidences of fertility have been reported in men with less severe forms of the syndrome.

In order to put this rather controversial evidence into perspective, Akhenaten should be pictured alongside his forebears and successors and the artistic conventions of the period should also be taken into account. Images of his grandfather, Tuthmosis IV (figure 44), and his father, Amenophis III (figure 45), depict similar physical attributes to Akhenaten himself. Both show the type of gynaecomastia characteristic of a hormonal imbalance although the association with schistosomiasis or obesity cannot be excluded. Smenkhkare and Tutankhamun (figure 46) also show this feminisation tendency. However the art of the period was characterised by a refinement of draftsmanship such that precise rendering of detail was combined with a softening of form and sensitivity of modelling which gave maximum expression to the subject. Akhenaten extended this style by revising the traditional proportions used to portray the human figure. Evidence is accruing that Smenkhkare and Tutankhamun were sons of Akhenaten (by a lesser wife, Kiya) and blood grouping has proved identical in both mummies. In addition, the body thought to be that of Smenkhkare revealed bones suggestive of hypogonadism with an arm span 11 cm greater than his height (the two measurements should be equal).

Derry, the anatomist who examined Tutankhamun's mummy in 1925,

47. (Right) Head of the infant Tutankhamun emerging from a lotus flower, Eighteenth Dynasty. (Courtesy of the Egyptian Museum, Cairo, JE 60723.)

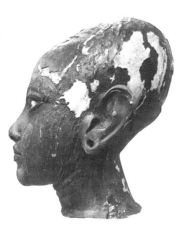

was surprised by the very unusual shape of the young Pharaoh's head, a feature of prominence on statues and paintings of the Amarna period (figure 47). In a later postmortem (Harrison, 1972), Tutankhamun's skull measurements were found to be within normal limits.

Both Smenkhkare and Tutankhamun were married to daughters of Akhenaten and Queen Nefertiti (Meretaten and Ankhsenpaaten respectively), and both died at about the same age without, as far as is known, producing offspring. However, two mummified female foetuses were found in Tutankhamun's tomb and, although serological analysis of one of the foetuses does not prove conclusively that Tutankhamun fathered the child, his name was on both caskets. The foetus was between thirty-six and forty weeks gestation and was still-born. It manifests multiple skeletal anomalies including scoliosis, spina bifida and the inheritable condition known as Sprengel's deformity (upward displacement of the scapula, in this case the left one, figure 48).

If Tutankhamun and Ankhsenpaaten *were* the parents of this unfortunate child, perhaps the end of the royal bloodline of the Eighteenth Dynasty owed more to an inheritance of the past than to a contemporary misfortune.

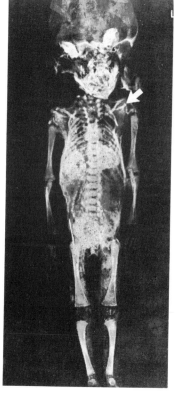

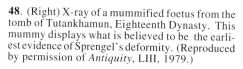

48. (Right) X-ray of a mummified foetus from the tomb of Tutankhamun, Eighteenth Dynasty. This mummy displays what is believed to be the earliest evidence of Sprengel's deformity. (Reproduced by permission of *Antiquity*, LIII, 1979.)

5
The medical papyri

In 1873 Georg Ebers, a German Egyptologist, acquired in Thebes a papyrus which had been discovered in a tomb in about 1860. Originally it was a roll 20.72 metres long but divided into pages of twenty lines each, totalling 108 columns, the scribe wrongly numbering them 110. The roll was cut up and bound in modern codex form and is now housed in the University of Leipzig (figure 49). The best known translation is by B. Ebbell, 1937. On the reverse are calendar notations which date its origin to about 1555 BC. It contains 876 remedies and mentions 500 substances used in medical treatment. 55 of the prescriptions feature urine and faeces as the main components. Excrement of lion, panther, ibex, gazelle and ostrich must have been extremely difficult to obtain in Egypt.

Like the other medical papyri, the Ebers Papyrus is wonderfully descriptive:

Flow away cold, son of the cold, who breaks the bones, who shatters the skull, so that sickness overtakes the seven openings in the head of the followers of Re, who appeal to Thoth in prayer. Behold I have used your medicine against you ... Milk of a woman who has given birth to a boy, and fragrant gum will get rid of you ... (Eb 763.)

The Ebers Papyrus describes treatment of and prescriptions for stomach complaints, coughs, colds, bites, head ailments and diseases; liver complaints, burns and other kinds of wounds; itching, complaints in fingers and toes; salves for wounds and pains in the veins, muscles and nerves; diseases of the tongue, toothache, ear pains, women's diseases; beauty preparations, household remedies against vermin, the two books about the heart and veins, and diagnosis for tumours.

The papyrus recommends the use of cauterisation to combat excessive bleeding. One type of lump described as 'a pocket full of gumwater' (perhaps an abscess or cyst) should be dealt with as follows: 'You should give it the cutting treatment; beware of the *mt* [blood vessel]' (Eb 871).

For a 'vessel-tumour' (this may not have been a blood vessel — the word *mt* or the plural *mtw* sometimes stood for hollow vessel; sometimes for solid strands such as tendons; the word for penis was also *mt*), the instructions are that such a tumour 'comes from a wound of the vessel. Then you should give it the cutting treatment. It (the knife) should be heated in the fire; the bleeding is not great' (Eb 872). So the actions of cutting and cauterising were carried out simultaneously and

49. A page from the Ebers Papyrus, New Kingdom. (Courtesy of the Universitätsbibliothek, Leipzig.)

the 'knife' must have been made of metal — copper or bronze. Egyptian copper contained natural deposits of arsenic which made it particularly hard and suitable for surgical blades. Further on in the papyrus is another untranslatable vessel-tumour — the *sft*. Here the physician is recommended to use 'the reed for cutting treatments' (Eb 571) and that 'if it bleeds a lot, you must burn it with fire'. In this case the knife was a far more readily available and disposable blade — the reed (figures 50

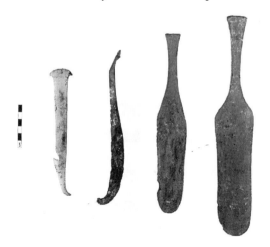

50. Four bronze knives from Gurob, Eighteenth to Nineteenth Dynasties. (Courtesy of the Petrie Museum of Egyptian Archaeology, University College London, UC 7748, 7749, 7779, 7745.)

51. The four words for 'knife'. The determinatives in (a), (b) and (c) represent the more common forms of flint or metal knives but the determinative in (d) refers to the reed or disposable blade sometimes used by Egyptian doctors. (Drawing by Helena Jaeschke.)

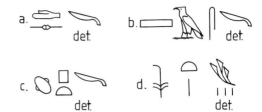

and 51). The instructions in the papyrus were most specific about when not to apply the knife. 'Serpentine windings' were not to be touched (varicose veins perhaps) because the result would be 'head on the ground' (Eb 876)!

In 1862 Edwin Smith, an American Egyptologist, bought a papyrus roll in Luxor. It was 4.67 metres long and 33.02 cm wide. On one side there are seventeen columns, each consisting of 77 lines, and the reverse has $4^{1}/_{2}$ columns of 92 lines each. It has been dated at about 1600 BC but Old Kingdom words in the text suggest that it was copied from a work written around 2500 BC, when the pyramids were being built (figure 52). It was published in 1930 with a translation and commentary by James Henry Breasted and is now housed in the New York Academy of Medicine.

52. Column XI of the Edwin Smith Papyrus; Second Intermediate Period but copied from an Old Kingdom text. (Courtesy of the New York Academy of Medicine.)

The Edwin Smith Papyrus contains descriptions of 48 surgical cases from the head to the thorax which are mostly traumatic in origin. Each case is given a title followed by a description of the method of examination. The diagnosis is preceded by one of three assessments: 'an ailment which I will treat'; 'an ailment with which I will contend'; 'an ailment not to be treated'. A description of the treatment is followed by a glossary explaining the meanings of Old Kingdom phrases to later readers. The Smith Papyrus contains what is probably the first description of the human brain:

> When you examine a man with a ... wound on his head, which
> goes to the bone; his skull is broken; broken open is the brain of
> his skull ... these windings which arise in poured metal. Some-
> thing is there ... that quivers (and) flutters under your fingers like
> the weak spot in the head of a child which has not yet grown hard
> ... Blood flows from his two nostrils. (S 6.)

But perhaps the most exciting sentences are to be found right at the
beginning of the papyrus:

> The counting of anything with the fingers (is done) to recognise
> the way the heart goes. There are vessels in it leading to every
> part of the body ... When a Sekhmet priest, any *sinw* doctor ...
> puts his fingers to the head ... to the two hands, to the place of the
> heart ... it speaks ... in every vessel, every part of the body. (S1.)

It is too fanciful to suggest that the Egyptians understood the relationship of the heart to the circulation of the blood — this was to be the
English physician William Harvey's great discovery in the early seven-
teenth century. However, they believed the heart to be the source of life
within the body and may, indeed, have felt the pulse and measured it by

53. The Kahun Medical Papyrus, Twelfth Dynasty. (Courtesy of the Petrie Museum of
Egyptian Archaeology, University College London, UC 32057.)

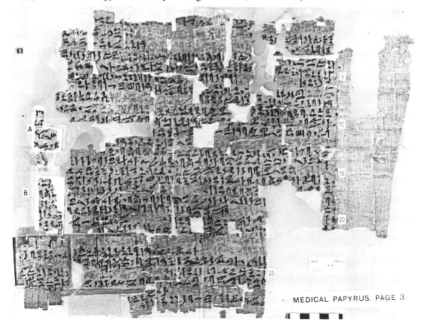

MEDICAL PAPYRUS. PAGE 3.

comparison with their own pulses.

The Egyptians also believed that all the 'inner juices of the body' flowed through vessels emanating from the heart and collected at the anus, whence they could again be redistributed to various parts of the body. Air, blood, urine, mucus, semen and faeces flowed around the system, usually in harmony, but occasionally getting out of hand and thence precipitating an illness.

The Kahun Medical Papyrus was found, with other Middle Kingdom papyri, by Petrie in the town of Kahun in 1889. Consisting of only three pages, it has been variously dated betweeen 2100 and 1900 BC. It is preserved in the Petrie Museum of Egyptian Archaeology at University College London (UC 32057, figure 53). The papyrus is devoted to diseases of women and pregnancy and is possibly the oldest medical papyrus to be discovered. It was first published in 1898 as a hieroglyphic transcript with a translation by F. Ll. Griffiths. A revised translation by John Stevens was published in 1975. Here are a few examples of the diagnoses and treatments of the world's earliest gynaecologists:

> Instructions for a woman whose womb has become diseased through journeying. You should proceed to ask her: 'What do you smell?'. If she answer, 'I smell fries', you should declare about her, 'This is a disorder of the womb'. You should prescribe for it; her fumigation over everything she smells as fries. (K 2.)

And possibly the first recorded case of rape:

> Instructions for a woman suffering in her vagina and likewise in every limb: one who has been maltreated. You should declare about her: 'This has bound up her womb.' You should prescribe for it; oil to be eaten until she is well. (K 9.)

In order to prevent conception the papyrus recommends 'excrement of crocodile dispersed finely in sour milk' (K 21) or '454 ml [sic] of honey injected into her vagina, with a pinch of natron' (K 22). In order to determine fertility, the following could be tried:

> You should have her sit upon a floor overlain with the lees of sweet ale, placing a mash of dates ... vomiting, she will give birth. Now concerning the number of each vomiting that comes out of her mouth, this is the number of child bearings ... However, should she not vomit, she will not give birth ever. (K 27.)

The Berlin Papyrus was discovered in a jar by Heinrich Brugsch during excavations at Saqqara in the early years of the twentieth century. It consists of 279 lines of prescriptions and has been dated around 1350-1200 BC. Translated and published by Walter Wreszinksi in 1909, it is housed in the Berlin Museum with a fifteen-column papyrus dealing with childbirth and infants and dated about 1550 BC. The Berlin Papyrus contains a test for pregnancy:

> Barley and emmer. The woman must moisten it with urine every day ... if both grow, she will give birth. If the barley grows, it means a male child. If the emmer grows, it means a female child.
> If neither grows, she will not give birth. (Bln 199.)

In 1963 Ghalioungui found that, whilst urine from non-pregnant women *prevented* the growth of (modern) barley and wheat, it proved impossible to detect the sex of an unborn child from the *rate* of growth of either grain. Nevertheless, the fact that the Egyptians recognised that urine carried the pregnancy factor was remarkable. The standardisation of reliable urine tests for pregnancy did not occur until 1929.

The Chester Beatty Papyrus VI, housed in the British Museum, is dated around 1200 BC and consists of eight columns dealing solely with diseases of the anus. It was translated and annotated by F. Jonckheere in 1947.

The Hearst Papyrus, now in the University of California, dates from about 1550 BC and appears to be the formulary of a practising physician. It is incomplete and contains eighteen columns. A translation by Walter Wreszinski of the Hearst Papyrus and the London Papyrus (*c.*1350 BC) was published in 1912. The Hearst Papyrus contains over 250 prescriptions and spells and has a section on bones and bites (notably the hippopotamus bite) and affections of the fingers. It also deals with tumours, burns, diseases of women, ears, eyes and teeth. The London Papyrus contains 61 recipes, only 25 of which are medical, the remainder being magical.

The Brooklyn Museum Papyri, translated in 1966-7 by Serge Sauneron, contain a mixture of magical and rational medicine, particularly with relation to birth and post-partum care. Also included in these papyri is a book of snakebites, describing all the possible snakes to be found in Egypt with a compendium of treatments.

The Carlsberg Papyrus Number VIII, translated by E. Iversen in 1939 and housed in the University of Copenhagen, deals mainly with eye diseases almost identical to those described in the Ebers Papyrus, and with obstetrics very similar to that in the Kahun, Berlin and Ebers Papyri.

The Ramesseum IV and V Papyri are of the same era as the Kahun Papyrus. A translation of both papyri by J. W. B. Barns was published in 1956. Papyrus IV is medico-religious and deals with obstetrics and gynaecology. Papyrus V is purely medical and deals mainly with stiffened limbs. The series of obstetric prescriptions and prognostications in the Carlsberg, Ebers, Berlin and Kahun Papyri are so similar that it is likely that they were all taken from the same source.

6
Drugs and the prescription

Of the many pieces of jewellery found in Tutankhamun's tomb, one of the richest was a massive gold bracelet. It was stored in the same cartouche-shaped box as his earrings, suggesting that it was a personal possession, worn by the Pharaoh in his lifetime, and not a funerary object. The central feature is a gold openwork scarab encrusted with lapis lazuli. Two identical botanical ornaments flank the scarab, each consisting of a mandrake fruit supported by two floral buds believed to be poppies (figure 54).

The mandrake (*Mandragora officinarum* L.), containing the narcotics atropine and scopolamine, grew prolifically in Palestine and was grown in Egypt from the New Kingdom onwards. It is a poisonous plant and when mixed with beer or wine it induces unconsciousness. The Egyptians believed that it possessed aphrodisiac properties and promoted conception (figure 55). In wall paintings of several Eighteenth Dynasty Theban tombs baskets of this fruit are represented, and men and women are sometimes depicted smelling or eating it at banquets (figure 56).

Many important raw materials used in the manufacture of medicines came from outside Egypt and, from Protodynastic times, trade exchange was a vital feature of Egyptian expansion. From Syria and Asia Minor came fir (*Abies cilicia* Carr.), its pungent resin invaluable as an antiseptic and an embalming material. Oil of fir was used as an anthelmintic (Eb 77) and to clean infected wounds (Eb 522b). From eastern Africa came aloe (*Aloe vera* L.), used to 'expel catarrh from the nose' (Eb 63), and cinnamon (*Cinnamonium zeylanicum* Nees), an essential ingredient in an unguent for ulcerated gums (Eb 553) and in incense. Cinnamon, frankincense and myrrh were brought back by Queen Hatshepsut's expedition from Punt during the New Kingdom. Punt was an important trade link in the chain of commerce which spread from Africa, the East and Europe.

Temple records of about 1200 BC reveal that in one year the temple of Amun in Thebes burned 2189 jars and 304,093 Egyptian bushels of incense. Incense was burned extensively in Egyptian homes and was used both to sweeten the air and as a fumigator (figure 57). The burning of incense produces phenol, or carbolic acid.

> ... to sweeten the smell of the house or clothes: dry myrrh, pignon, frankincense, rush-nut, bark of cinnamon, reed from Phoenicia, liquid styrax, are ground fine, mixed together and a little thereof is placed over a fire. (Eb 852.)

Other fumigators included fleabane (*Inula graveolens; Inula conyza*),

56

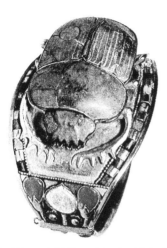
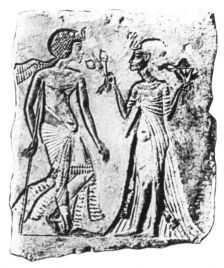

54. (Above left) Bracelet of gold, lapis lazuli, turquoise, carnelian and quartz found in the tomb of Tutankhamun. The design depicts a mandrake fruit flanked by poppies. Eighteenth Dynasty. (Courtesy of the Egyptian Museum, Cairo, JE 62360.)

55. (Above right) Painted sandstone relief showing Princess Meretaten offering a mandrake plant to her husband, Smenkhkare, Eighteenth Dynasty. (Courtesy of the State Museum, Berlin.)

56. (Below) Wall painting of ladies at a banquet. The girl second from right is offering a mandrake fruit to her companion (far right) and both are wearing lumps of perfume-impregnated fat on top of their wigs. From the tomb of Nebamun and Ipuky, Eighteenth Dynasty. (Courtesy of the Trustees of the British Museum, London, 37986.)

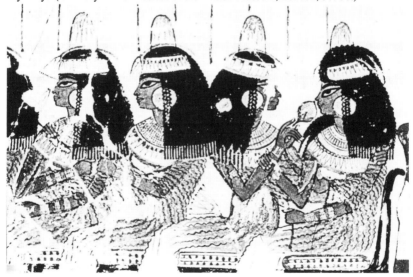

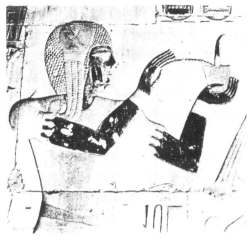

57. (Left) Painted wall relief depicting Seti I offering burning incense to Osiris. From the temple of Seti I, Abydos, Nineteenth Dynasty. (Photograph by the author.)

58. (Below) Determinatives meaning (a) mineral, (b) plant and (c) herb. These determinatives identify the root source of drugs and medicines. (Drawing by Helena Jaeschke.)

a   b   c

which is strongly antibacterial and was used, as the name suggests, to drive fleas from the house, and sulphur wort (*Peucedanum galbaniflora; Peucedanum officinale*), a fragrant gum resin imported from Persia and known in Egypt as 'green incense'.

Medicinal plants not native to Egypt were introduced during the Dynastic Period and continue to flourish to the present day. Henna (*Lawsonia inermis* L.; *Lawsonia alba* L.) probably originated from Persia but was grown in Egypt from the Late Period and probably earlier. The word *hnw* occurs in a prescription to treat hair loss (Eb 774) although whether henna was used to colour the hair is disputed. The pomegranate (*Punica granatum* L.) was introduced into Egypt during the New Kingdom, presumably from south-west Asia. Apart from its importance as a food, the root (which contains tannin) was used to dislodge roundworm (Eb 50).

Many words for plants cannot be translated from inscriptions and the papyri, and it must be assumed that they have not yet been identified. In addition, the Egyptian artist's rendering of a flower, shrub or tree was in many cases stylistic rather than representational. Some drugs and medicines would be unrecognisable without determinatives to identify the root source, which was generally of mineral, plant or herbal origin (figure 58).

A prescription in the Ebers Papyrus reads: 'powder of green pigment … grind to fine powder; bind upon it' (Eb 766). Green was an important colour to the Egyptians, probably because it was synonymous with the fruitfulness of the land and its rebirth after the annual inundation. In most cases, 'green' referred to one particular green stone — malachite.

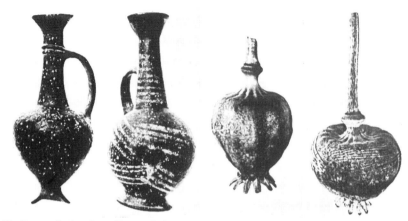

59. Pottery juglets from Cyprus (left two) which were probably used for carrying opium mixed with wine or water. The sizes (about 11.5 cm high) and shapes compare with poppy capsules (right two), Eighteenth Dynasty. (From G. Majno; *The Healing Hand: Man and Wound in the Ancient World.* Cambridge [Mass] Harvard University Press, 1975, figure 3.21. Reproduced by permission of *Antiquity*.)

This is copper carbonate and was found in the Eastern Desert and on the Sinai peninsula. Another 'green' was chrysocolla, copper silicate, which has a touch of blue. A cheaper 'green' was made by grinding into a powder a glass made by melting sand with natron and copper minerals. This green pigment was used in ointments to cleanse wounds and also as an eye paint used both as a decoration and to prevent the eye diseases so common in Egypt (cover illustration).

Copper does, to an appreciable extent, prevent the penetration of bacteria, particularly *staphylococci*. Black pigment was also used as an eye make-up and a salve and the Egyptians called this *msdmt*. *Msdmt* is lead sulphide or 'galena' which was mined in the Eastern Desert at Quseir el-Qadim on the Red Sea coast. There is little evidence to suggest that the use of galena resulted in lead toxicity. Indeed, data from geochemical measurements and analysis of 105 Nubian bodies (*c*.3300 BC to *c*.AD 750) from the Scandinavian Joint Expedition to Sudanese Nubia during 1960-4 have estimated the lead intake of ancient Egyptians to be about one hundred times less than that of modern man.

The Edwin Smith Papyrus contains a drug referred to as *spn*, which cautiously translates as 'poppy' (*Papaver somniferum* L.), the plant whose alkaloids produce opium and morphine. A remedy for a crying child is given in the Ebers papyrus: '... *spn* seeds, fly dung from the wall, is made to a paste, strained and drunk for four days. The crying will cease instantly' (Eb 782). Although *Papaver somniferum* (and *Papaver rhoeas* L.) were grown in Egypt from the middle of the Eighteenth Dynasty, it was during this period that small jugs were imported from Cyprus and Syria of comparable size, shape and colour to poppy capsules, some even bearing parallel lines which suggested the slits made in the capsules to extract the potent sap. It is almost certain that these exquisite containers were used to export the costly drug opium, dissolved in wine or water (figure 59).

In five hundred prescriptions and remedies, an important constituent is honey. Honey is highly resistant to bacterial growth. It is extremely hypertonic and draws water from bacterial cells, causing them to shrivel and die. It also has an antibiotic action due to the presence of inhibine, a bactericidal enzyme secreted by the pharyngeal glands of the bee.

In modern studies honey has proven to be effective against *staphylococcus*, *salmonella* and *candida* bacteria and has been used to treat surgical wounds, burns and ulcers, having more rapid healing qualities than conventional treatment. Another bee product called propolis (bee glue) is a hard, resinous material derived by bees from plant juices. Like honey, propolis also has antibiotic as well as preservative properties and is used by bees to seal cracks in their hives and to deal with foreign 'invaders'. The perfectly preserved body of a small mouse, which crept into an ancient Egyptian hive three thousand years ago, was found, covered with propolis, dried out and with no sign of decomposition.

The beautiful ibis bird was sacred to the Egyptians, being the incarnation of Thoth, god of the scribes (figure 60). They believed that the ibis, standing in the shallows of the Nile, filled its long beak with water and introduced it into its anus, squirting in the water and flushing out its insides. Marshmallow (*Althea* species), hemp (*Cannabis sativa* L.), melon leaves (*Cucumis melo* L.), cumin (*Cumin cyminum* L.), moringa oil (*Moringa pterygosperma; Moringa aptera*), bean meal (*Vigna sinensis* L.) and zizyphus (*Zizyphus spina-Christi* Willd) were all used in prescriptions for enemas or to 'cool the anus'.

One of the seven medical papyri and 81 prescriptions refer only to the anus. The Egyptians considered the faeces to contain a horrific substance they called *whdw*, roughly translated as 'the rots'. Despite this, mud and excrement were included in many medicaments, but treating 'like with like' was a practice not unknown in ancient and medieval medicine and is the basis of homeopathic medicine today.

As *whdw* travelled all over the body and turned up in suppurating sores, ulcers and wounds, it might have seemed natural to give it a taste of its own medicine, and in some cases it did indeed work. In the mid nineteenth century Louis Pasteur discovered that certain substances

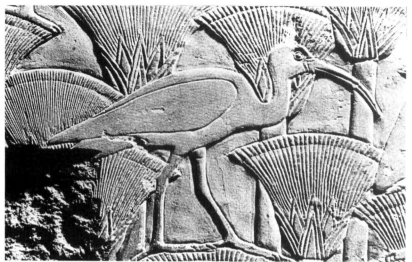

60. Painted limestone wall relief of an ibis, whose long beak and preening behaviour led to the invention of the enema. From the funerary temple of Userkaf, Saqqara, Fifth Dynasty. (Courtesy of the Egyptian Museum, Cairo, JE 56601.)

produced by micro-organisms have an antimicrobial action of their own. Bacteria living in the bodies of humans or animals release their excretory products into the faeces and urine, which become a source of antibiotic substances. Certain soils do indeed produce fungi which have a destructive effect upon specific bacteria. Aureomycin, discovered in 1948, was extracted from soil and proved to be particularly effective in the treatment of trachoma. Modern cephalosporin antibiotics are descended from an original species of *Cephalosporium* isolated from a sewage outfall in Sardinia in 1945.

The various prescriptions often mention beer as an agent by which many drugs were to be administered and the Egyptians drank a large amount of beer. But they knew and used the benefits of yeast, applying it raw to boils and ulcers and swallowing it to soothe digestive disorders. Yeast contains vitamin B as well as antibiotic agents which are particularly effective against the agents of furunculosis.

A royal physician named Iwty, who lived in the time of the New Kingdom and possibly attended Ramesses I, had a special pharmacy for preparing medicines. Many doctors discovered their own remedies or had them handed down from their fathers or teachers and these were jealously guarded. A remedy prescribed by a doctor was sometimes issued in a container with the prescription written on it. It was not until modern times that the physician became divorced from the actual preparation of his own medicines. For those he prepared himself, maybe with herbs he gathered personally, he would have direct knowledge of their formulation (figure 61). His other medicines would have been made by an apothecary known to him and probably to his special direction. Consequently a doctor often gained his reputation by the potency of his brew.

In the course of discovering which drugs were efficacious and which were lethal, and to what proportions components performed best in a medicament, the Egyptians developed the prescription. They weighed and measured this prescription carefully in a most novel way. Fractions were expressed by dissecting the eye of the god Horus, the son of Isis and Osiris, which was torn out and ripped to pieces by his evil brother, Seth (figure 62). Today we use the character R to designate the word 'prescription' — a direct descendant of the symbol for the 'Eye of Horus'.

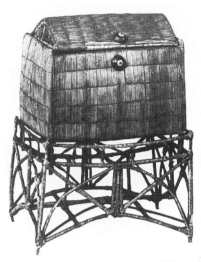

61. A pharmacist's carrying case, Eleventh Dynasty. (Courtesy of the State Museum, Berlin, 1176.)

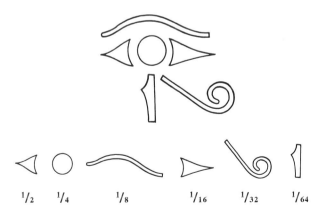

$$^1/_2 \qquad ^1/_4 \qquad ^1/_8 \qquad ^1/_{16} \qquad ^1/_{32} \qquad ^1/_{64}$$

62. The eye of Horus with, below it, the hieroglyphs for the fractions of the prescription (eye of Horus). (Drawings by the author.)

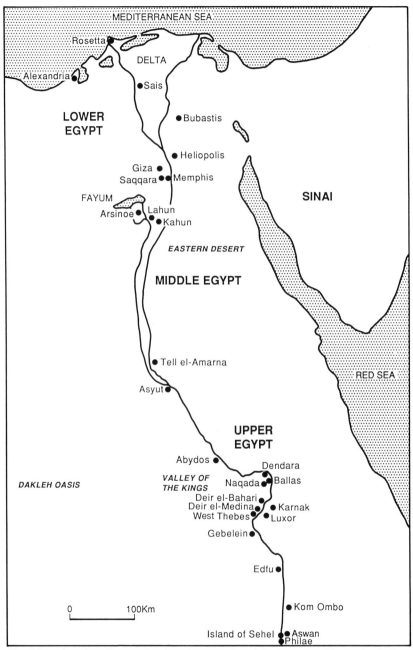

63. Map of ancient Egypt, showing sites mentioned in the text. (Drawn by Robert Dizon.)

7
Glossary of medical terms

Abscess: a collection of pus in a cavity produced by tissue disintegration and displacement.

Abscess, dental: an abscess, often close to the root of a tooth, which destroys bone and adjoining soft tissues.

Achondroplasia: short-limbed dwarfism due to a dominant genetic mutation.

Acromegaly: a chronic disease marked by enlargement of the hands, feet and bones of the head and chest. It is caused by excessive secretion, or sensitivity to growth hormone developing in adult life.

Alveolar bone: the part of the bone of the jaw to which the teeth are attached.

Anthelmintic: a remedy for infestation with worms.

Anthracosis: blackening of the lungs due to deposits of carbon particles.

Aorta: the main arterial trunk of the body.

Appendicular adhesions: bands of tissue produced as a result of inflammation of the appendix and which unite those surrounding parts which normally are separate.

Arteriosclerosis: narrowing and hardening of the lumen of the arteries.

Arthritis: inflammation of a joint.

Ascites: abnormal accumulation of a fluid in the abdominal cavity.

Atheromatous: affected with or pertaining to atheroma (the process affecting blood vessels which involves the formation of cholesterol deposits which later become fibrotic or calcified).

Calcification: the deposition of calcareous matter within organic tissue so that it becomes hardened.

Carcinoma: a malignant tumour originating in epithelial cells. These cells cover the external surface of the entire body and line all hollow structures within the body with the exception of blood and lymphatic vessels.

Cataract: opacity in the crystalline lens of the eye.

Cauterisation: the act of burning tissue to stop bleeding.

Cervical spine: that part of the spine related to the neck.

Cholecystitis: inflammation of the gall bladder.

Cholelithiasis: the formation of stones in the gall bladder.

Cirrhosis: a chronic progressive inflammation of the liver associated with distortion, toughening and atrophy.

Cleft palate: a congenital fissure in the midline of the hard palate.

Conjunctivitis: inflammation of the conjunctiva (the mucous membrane lining the eyelids and anterior surface of the eyeball).

Cretinism: a congenital thyroid dysfunction producing physical and mental retardation.

Dental attrition: the process of wearing down the biting surfaces of the teeth by mastication.

Dental caries: invasion of the tooth substance by micro-organisms; associated with dietary sugars.

Dysplasia: abnormal development of tissue.

Endoscope: an instrument for examining the interior of a hollow organ.

Eunuchoid: term applied to a male in whom the testes have not developed or where the external genitals may be complete but the internal secretion is lacking.

Fibroadenoma: a tumour in which there is dense formation of fibrous tissue.

Furunculosis: a condition of being affected by furuncles or boils.

Galactagogue: an agent which increases the secretion or flow of milk.

Gynaecomastia: a condition in the male in which the mammary glands are excessively developed.

Haematuria: the presence of blood in the urine.

Halitosis: fetid or offensive breath.

Hernia: protrusion of abdominal contents through the abdominal wall.

Hernia, scrotal: hernia of the groin which has descended into the scrotum.

Histology: the branch of biological science which is concerned with the anatomy of tissues and their microscopic cellular structure.

Hydatid: a cystic stage in the life cycle of the parasite *Echinococcus granulosis.*

Hydrocephalus: an abnormal increase of cerebrospinal fluid within the skull.

Hypertonic solution: a solution which exerts an osmotic pressure.

Hypertrophy: an increase in the number or size of the cells of which a tissue is composed as a result of increase in function of that tissue.

Infantile megacolon: a condition, usually congenital, in which there is a great dilatation of part or the whole of the large intestine.

Keratosis senilis: a lesion of the skin seen in elderly people.

Kyphosis: the excessive forward curvature of the spine.

Lactose: the natural sugar found in milk.

Leucoma: a white scar of the cornea.

Meningioma: a benign tumour of the meninges (the covering or sheaths of the brain and spinal cord).

Mitral valve: the valve separating the left atrium from the left ventricle in the heart.

Naevus: any birthmark or localised abnormality of developmental origin.

Narcotic: a drug which induces a stuporous condition or sleep.

Osmotic: relating to osmosis (the movement of a solvent across a membrane to an area where there is a higher concentration of solution to which the membrane is impermeable).

Osteo-arthritis: chronic arthritis of a degenerative type associated with age or trauma.

Osteocartilaginous exostosis: an outgrowth made up of bone and cartilage extending from the surface of a bone.

Osteochondroma: a tumour composed of both bony and cartilaginous tissues.

Osteomyelitis: inflammation of the interior of a bone, especially affecting the marrow spaces.

Osteoporosis: rarefaction of bone.

Osteosarcoma: a malignant tumour of bone cells.

Pathogenesis: the mode of origin and development of diseased conditions.

Periodontal disease: inflammation and eventual erosion of the structures surrounding a tooth.

Periostitis: inflammation of the periosteum (the connective tissue covering of bone).

Pleurisy: inflammation of the pleura (the membrane which covers the lungs).

Pneumothorax: the presence of air within the thorax, resulting in partial or complete collapse of the lung.

Poliomyelitis: acute inflammation of the anterior horn cells of the spinal cord due to an enterovirus infection which may result in paralysis of the limbs.

Polydactyly: the presence of more than the normal number of fingers or toes.

Prolapse: the sinking down or protrusion of a part of the body or organ.

Pseudohermaphroditism: a congenital condition in which the gonads are either testes or ovaries but the external genitals are either characteristic of the opposite sex or a mixture of both male and female.

Psoas muscle: the long muscle which flexes the hip joint, extending from the lumbar vertebrae to the femur.

Rickets: a disturbance of the calcium/phosphorus metabolism in the growing child as a result of vitamin D deficiency.

Sacral erosion: destruction of the sacrum (the composite bone formed by the fusion of the sacral vertebrae, forming the back of the pelvis).

Sacro-iliac joint: the joint formed between the sacrum and the ileum in the pelvis.

Sand pneumoconiosis: a disease of the respiratory tract caused by the inhalation of particles of sand.

Scapula: shoulder blade.

Schistosomiasis: a group of diseases caused by trematode parasitic flukes of the family Schistosomatidae. They live in the veins of various internal organs and lay eggs which reach the exterior mainly by the urine or faeces.

Scoliosis: lateral curvature of the spine.

Serology: the medical science which is concerned with the study of blood sera, identifying group-specific substances, proteins and enzymes.

Smallpox: a generalised virus infection with a vesicular rash (variola).

Solar keratosis: a lesion of the skin seen in elderly people with long-continued exposure to the sun.

Spina bifida: a defect in development of the vertebral column with variable protrusion of the contents of the spinal canal through the gap.

Splenomegaly: enlargement of the spleen.

Squamous: resembling a scale; platelike.

Squamous cell papilloma: a stalked (skin) tumour lined with squamous cells.

Talipes equinovarus: club foot.

Temporomandibular joint: the joint which connects and articulates the temporal bone and the mandible in the skull.

Tendo Achilles: the tendon which joins the calf muscle to the heel. It is used extensively in walking, running and jumping.

Tetraplegia: paralysis of both arms and legs.

Tibia: the long bone between the knees and ankle joints.

Tomography: body-section radiography. A radiographic technique which shows images of structures lying in a predetermined plane of tissue, while blurring out by movement the images of the structures in other planes, above or below.

Trachoma: an eye infection caused by *Chlamydia trachomatis*. Untreated, it can lead to blindness.

Ulcer: a lesion of the skin or mucous surface in which the superficial cells are destroyed and deeper tissues exposed in an open sore.

Vascular: pertaining to a blood vessel or vessels.

Vesicovaginal fistula: a communication between the bladder and the vagina.

8
Further reading

The books listed in this section have been selected because of their particular interest. In addition, there are many general books on Egyptology which contain sections on Egyptian medicine. Some of the books listed below are now out of print although they may occasionally be found in good second-hand and specialist antiquarian bookshops.

There are societies for the study of the history of medicine in most major cities of the world, many of which have excellent libraries. In the United Kingdom there are several libraries specialising in the history of medicine. The Wellcome Institute for the History of Medicine, the Royal College of Physicians and the Royal Society of Medicine (all in London) have important historical collections and, whilst these libraries are not generally open to the public, it may be possible to obtain reader's tickets for the purposes of specific research.

Aldred, Cyril. *Akhenaten, King of Egypt.* Thames and Hudson, 1986.

Breasted, J. H. *The Edwin Smith Papyrus* (two volumes). The University of Chicago Press, 1930.

Brothwell, D. R., and Chiarelli, B. A. (editors). *Population Biology of the Ancient Egyptians.* Academic Press, 1973.

Brothwell, D., and Higgs, E. *Science in Archaeology.* Thames and Hudson, second edition, 1969.

Bryan, Cyril P. *The Papyrus Ebers with an Introduction by Professor G. Elliot Smith.* Geoffrey Bles, 1930.

David, A. Rosalie. *The Pyramid Builders of Ancient Egypt — A Modern Investigation of Pharaoh's Workforce.* Guild Publishing, 1986.

Ebbell, B. *The Papyrus Ebers, The Greatest Egyptian Medical Document.* Levin and Munksgaard, Copenhagen, 1937.

Gardiner, Sir A. 'Hieratic Papyri in the British Museum' in Sir A. Gardiner (editor), *Chester Beatty Gift*, British Museum, 1935.

Gardiner, Sir A. *Egyptian Grammar.* Oxford University Press, 1950.

Gardiner, Sir A. *The Ramesseum Papyri.* Oxford University Press, 1955.

Kamal, Hassan. *Dictionary of Pharaonic Medicine.* The National Publication House, Cairo, 1967.

Leca, Ange-Pierre. *La Médecine Égyptienne au Temps des Pharaons.* Roger Dacosta, Paris, 1983.

Lucas, A. *Ancient Egyptian Materials and Industries.* Edward Arnold, fourth edition, 1962.

Majno, G. *The Healing Hand: Man and Wound in the Ancient World.*

Harvard University Press, Cambridge (Massachusetts), 1975. This book has an excellent bibliography.

Manniche, Lise. *Sexual Life in Ancient Egypt*. KPI, 1987.

Manniche, Lise. *An Ancient Egyptian Herbal*. British Museum Publications, 1989.

Nunn, J. F. *Ancient Egyptian Medicine*. British Museum Press, 1996.

Ruffer, M. A. *The Paleopathology of Ancient Egypt*. Chicago University Press, 1921.

Sauneron, Serge. 'The Wilbour Papyri in Brooklyn: a Progress Report', *The Brooklyn Museum Annual X, 1968-1969*. 1969, pages 109-15.

Singer, Charles, and Ashworth Underwood, E. *A Short History of Medicine*. Clarendon Press, Oxford, second edition, 1962.

Thorwald, Jürgen. *Science and Secrets of Early Medicine*. Thames and Hudson, 1962.

9
Museums

The following museums contain medical and related exhibits. In addition, some universities and medical institutes preserve medical papyri and artefacts which, although not generally available for public viewing, may be accessible to students and researchers. Some of these institutions are acknowledged in the legends to figures.

United Kingdom

Ashmolean Museum of Art and Archaeology, Beaumont Street, Oxford OX1 2PH. Telephone: 01865 278000. Website: www.ashmol.ox.ac.uk

The British Museum, Great Russell Street, London WC1B 3DG. Telephone: 020 7636 1555. Website: www.thebritishmuseum.ac.uk

Liverpool Museum, William Brown Street, Liverpool L3 8EN. Telephone: 0151 478 4399. Website: www.nmgm.org.uk

Manchester Museum, The University of Manchester, Oxford Road, Manchester M13 9PL. Telephone: 0161 275 2634. Website: www.museum.man.ac.uk

Petrie Museum of Egyptian Archaeology, University College London, Gower Street, London WC1E 6BT. Telephone: 020 7679 2884. Website: www.petrie.ucl.ac.uk

Science Museum, Exhibition Road, South Kensington, London SW7 2DD. Telephone: 020 7942 4000. Website: www.sciencemuseum.org.uk

Belgium

Musées Royaux d'Art et d'Histoire, Avenue J. F. Kennedy, 1040 Brussels.

Canada

Museum of the History of Medicine, 288 Bloor Street West, Toronto M5S 1V8, Ontario.

Denmark

Ny Carlsberg Glyptotek, Dantes Plads, DK-1550 Copenhagen V.

Egypt

Egyptian Antiquities Museum, Tahrir Square, Cairo.

France

Musée du Louvre, Palais du Louvre, F-75041 Paris.

Germany
Ägyptisches Museum, Schlosstrasse 70, 1000 Berlin 19.
Roemer-Pelizaeus Museum, Amsteiner 1, 3200 Hildesheim.

Holland
Rijksmuseum van Oudheden, Rapenburg 28, 2311 EW Leiden.

Italy
Museo Archeologico, Via della Colonna 96, Florence.

United States of America
The Brooklyn Museum, 200 Eastern Parkway, Brooklyn, New York, NY 11238.
Field Museum of Natural History, Roosevelt Road at Lakeshore Drive, Chicago, Illinois 60605.
University of Chicago Oriental Institute Museum, 1155 East 58th Street, Chicago, Illinois 60637.
Metropolitan Museum of Art, 5th Avenue at 82nd Street, New York, NY 10028.